ARTIFICIAL INSEMINATION BY DONOR

ARTIFICIAL INSEMINATION BY DONOR

a study of ethics, medicine, and law in our technological society

PHYLLIS CREIGHTON

Task Force on Human Life
The Anglican Church of Canada

The Anglican Book Centre
Toronto, Canada

Published by
The Anglican Book Centre
600 Jarvis Street
Toronto, Ontario
Canada M4Y 2J6

ISBN 0-919030-21-1

CONTENTS

PREFACE

This report has been prepared through the work of the Task Force on Human Life. The Task Force was established in January 1972, at the request of the February 1971 General Synod, to study ethical issues being posed by medicine and the life sciences. In its interim report to General Synod Quebec 1975, the Task Force noted that it had begun a study of A.I.D. It sought permission then to write a full report whose purpose would be

> to provide insights and guidance to help the persons involved in making responsible choices — the men and women facing the dilemmas of unwished for sterility, the doctors wishing to adopt a responsible approach to newly available medical techniques, the lawyers whose counsel might be sought, the legislators who ultimately will have to deal with the complex problems the techniques raise. As in its report on abortion, the Task Force wishes to promote serious discussion and to aid the church and community to make responsible decisions in this expanding area of medical science.

General Synod authorized it to complete its work and to submit the report to the National Executive Council for subsequent circulation (R 38). It is with these purposes in view, and in response to General Synod's resolution, that this study has been written.

Members of the Task Force on Human Life, for this study, 1973-77

The Most Rev. E. W. Scott, B.A., D.D., D.C.L., Primate.

The Rev. Canon Paul Chidwick, S.T.B., M.A. (Phil.), B.D., chairman, Task Force;
parish priest, St Mary's, Walkerville, Diocese of Huron.

Phyllis Creighton, M.A. (Hist.),
researcher, editor, *Dictionary of Canadian Biography*,
University of Toronto Press;
leader, marriage and family life education,
Diocese of Toronto.

The Rev. Canon Eugene Fairweather, M.A., Th.D., D.D.,
Keble professor of divinity, Trinity College,
University of Toronto.

The Rev. Charles R. Feilding, B.A., S.T.D.
(resigned from the Task Force, 1974)
professor emeritus of moral theology,
Trinity College, University of Toronto.

The Rev. Paul Gibson, B.A., L.Th.,
consultant in theological and continuing education,
Anglican Church of Canada.

Betty Graham, M.A. (Phil), M.S.W., D.S.L.,
former director of child welfare;
now director, York-Peel district,
Ministry of Community and Social Services, Ontario.

Melville G. Kerr, M.D.,
obstetrician and gynecologist;
professor at McMaster University 1973-74,
the University of Edinburgh 1974-77;
now chairman and professor, obstetrics
and gynecology, University of Calgary.

Stewart Kingstone, Q.C.
Lancaster, Mix, Welch, Kingstone,
Reed & Thorsteinson, St Catharines, Ontario.

David McCallion, M.A., Ph.D.,
professor of anatomy,
McMaster University, Hamilton, Ontario.

The Rev. E. James Reed, Ph.D.,
(resigned from the Task Force, June 1974)
professor of pastoral theology and psychology,
Trinity College, University of Toronto.

The Rev. Richard Roach, S.J., Ph.D., B.Th.,
professor of moral theology,
Regis College, Toronto;
presently at Marquette University, Wisconsin.

Thomas B. Robson, M.D., F.R.C.S. (C),
obstetrician and gynecologist,
Windsor, Ontario.

Cope Schwenger, M.D., D.P.H.,
professor of community health practice,
University of Toronto.

W. Stuart Ellis, LL.B., Q.C.,
St Catharines, Ontario.

FOREWORD

In the latter half of the 20th century man is discovering and learning to use God-given capacities to explore all aspects of existence — physical, personal and social — at radically deeper levels. His disciplined exploration has led to an explosion of knowledge which confronts individuals and society with new possibilities for action in a wide variety of realms. The decisions which are being and will be made in the face of the new possibilities almost always have moral and ethical dimensions, although these may not readily be recognized.

I am convinced that groups such as the Christian Church, with a primary concern about moral and ethical decision making must grapple with the implications of potential new courses of action as soon as these become feasible. Unfortunately, all too often in the past, practice has already become established before the moral issues involved have been examined in depth. It is my hope that the Church will reach the point of being able to think ahead and to give moral leadership rather than "tagging along" and often reacting negatively.

This report is an attempt to do this in a realm where new knowledge has made possible a course of action which matches the felt needs of some individuals in our society — the use of the now widely available technique of artificial insemination of a woman who desires children but whose husband is either infertile or genetically at risk in fathering a child and who therefore desires sperm provided by a donor.

The factors involved in studying this subject are complex. Our report does not pretend to be exhaustive, nor does it give ready-made answers. It is an attempt to identify and reflect upon some of the moral and ethical issues and to make possible more informed decision making. We know such issues arouse deep emotions, honest concern and even anxiety, and strong differences of opinion. We believe that these issues will not go away nor ought they to be ignored — rather they should be faced frankly, in a constant search for deeper knowledge of "the truth." So we hope that our report may lead others to explore, trusting in our Lord's promise that "Ye shall know the truth and the truth will make you free."

Edward Scott,
Primate

THE PROBLEM

Couples

You are young . . . eager for life. You would love a baby in your arms. But your husband had to have radiation therapy to control cancer. He is sterile. And the adoption agencies will only accept you as a foster parent.

Because of serious problems you had to have lengthy psychiatric treatment. You long for a baby. But your husband is not very fertile and hasn't been able to make you pregnant. You tried to adopt a baby. But the adoption agency has very few available. And, although you are now well and the psychiatrist expresses confidence, the agency will consider you only for adoption of an older child.

What do you do? Artificial insemination donor is a technique in which the seminal fluid of an anonymous donor is mechanically introduced into a woman's vagina in the hopes of producing conception. It was first employed nearly 100 years ago and has been used with increasing frequency for the past 30 years to give babies to women with such problems.[1] Is A.I.D. a good way for you to meet your needs? What are the risks in it? Is it legal? Morally right? Will it bring happiness?

These are real life problems which the Task Force on Human Life met in its study of A.I.D. Its concern for this aspect of medical care was stimulated by the request of member M.G. Kerr, an obstetrician and gynecologist, who wanted the group to share the perplexities he was encountering in his practice and to reach greater clarity about its complex ethical, medical, legal and social aspects. A.I.D. is being undertaken widely in Canada, in Vancouver, Calgary, Winnipeg, London, Hamilton, St. Catharines, Kitchener, Thunder Bay, Toronto, Ottawa, Montreal, Halifax. Thus A.I.D. is becoming a problem of interest not just to a handful of physicians but to society as a whole, and should be given informed study by both medical profession and public. A combination of changes in needs, attitudes and awareness underly the new situation.

Current needs and attitudes

10 to 12% of couples are thought to be infertile, and experts variously estimate that the man is wholly responsible for the infertility in from 10 to 50% of such couples.[2] Thus considerable numbers of people are unable to procreate the children they want. Until recently, adoption was an acceptable and available solution for such couples. However, in the last few years the situation has changed dramatically. Increased access to both effective contraceptives and sterilization, as well as resort to legalized abortion, have sharply reduced unplanned births.[3] There is also greater community acceptance of the single mother and so more unwed mothers are choosing to raise their children. There are thus far fewer infants available for adoption.[4] More successful counselling of troubled families, and preventive services, have also reduced the numbers of children removed from their parents and legally free for adoption.

The issue of adoption has another complex angle. There has been some growth in the practice of adopting children of other countries, such as Vietnam, Bangladesh, Korea and Ecuador. International Social Service and Families for Children (founded in Montreal a few years ago by a Unitarian minister) both handle such adoptions, with initial study of the prospective parents' home being undertaken by local Children's Aid Societies.[5] Delicate issues are involved — for instance the proud desire of other nations to take care of their own children and the difficulties of raising children of a different race — and time-consuming practical negotiations are also required. Such adoption appeals strongly to some Christians, especially to those with personal knowledge of another land or a deep concern for conditions abroad. They see it as a caring response to the needs of the children of the world. In our Task Force, the Reverend Charles Feilding particularly urged that this solution to the problems of childless couples should be taken seriously. Asserting that "the obligation to adopt abandoned children should be brought to the attention of married couples and should be seen and stated as a purpose of the institution of marriage," he held "it is nonsense to argue that there is a shortage of adoptable children when the shortage is created by law and provoked by international conflict; the shortage is artificial not real."[6]

Adoption is, however, in fact no longer a readily available solution for many couples.

At the same time, the climate of opinion appears to have been shifting from hostile rejection and disapproval of donor insemination to greater and more positive interest in the whole idea. This may be related to changes during the past decade in public attitudes on questions of sexual behaviour.[7] Media publicity has fostered public knowledge and acceptance of A.I.D. [8] The medical profession is slowly accepting that A.I.D. is a responsible form of treatment which should be available and professional bodies such as the British Medical Association (Peel Panel 1973) and the American Fertility Society have approved it as a medical procedure in recent years.[9] Closer to home, by 1974 it appeared in the fee schedule of the Ontario Medical Association, and in May 1975 the British Columbia Royal Commission on Family and Children's Law issued a favourable report on it.

In our society parenthood is becoming increasingly a deliberate choice, and while young couples in growing numbers seem to be choosing to be childless, most of us are sympathetic to the right of married couples to bear children, a right the United Nations' Universal Declaration of Human Rights indeed affirms. Although there is serious concern about the world's population crisis, few would want to use this ground to deprive the childless of medical help to solve their problem. Many of us are anxious about the increasing breakdown of marriages and families and the cynicism about their future; we are also seriously concerned about the promiscuity evident in our society; all this makes us more open to the longings of mature couples for children, and inclined to be supportive. It seems likely that doctors will be expected to meet people's needs by available techniques. Other technological developments — the growth of human semen cryobanking, of expert infertility investigation, and of concern for disabilities and diseases of genetic origin for which donor insemination might be an answer — are also conducing to increased use of A.I.D.

The couple's situation

The Task Force interviewed the couples mentioned at the beginning of this report, after they had reached the decision to have A.I.D. We would like to tell you something of their motivations, feelings and attitudes, as background for our discussion of the ethical issues involved in A.I.D.

When they became aware of their own infertility, both couples had turned first to the possibility of adoption. Neither husbands nor wives had felt it was imperative for her, as a woman, to bear a child; caring for a baby was what seemed important.

To the husband who had become sterile through life-saving medical treatment, adoption or A.I.D. were equally desirable, and although neither shared it with parents, his wife felt secure enough about A.I.D. that she was able to discuss feelings and prospects with a girl friend. They had to struggle with real uncertainties about his health and with the prospect he might die, but they opted to believe in their proven ability to cope with crises and to take this step with hope and faith in the future, trusting that, should need arise, friends and families would give support.

But for the other husband, coming to the choice of A.I.D. was a real struggle. Adopting a child "outside the two of us" seemed easier at first and the donor insemination she had begun to think of seemed a bad choice to him. They had already gone through several years of medical treatment for infertility, with disappointment and longing. When the adoption agency refused their application for a baby and offered an older child who would be able to protest that the mother was unfit if she again had personal problems, they felt they were treated with impersonal distrust and little consideration. With some fear, but feeling it was the only door open, he turned to A.I.D. He had to struggle then with deep feelings that the child would come from "her egg but not my sperm"; feelings of inequality and of being put down; feelings that a virile man could father a child, and resistance to sharing any part of the role a virile man should have. Intellectually he knew that the biological role in conception was only one aspect of fathering; so he struggled not to blow it up out of proportion, to accept that life was imperfect and he had the weakness of infertility, to think about the fact that his wife would fully experience motherhood and to come to the belief that he would be able to get over the baby's not being "his child," over not being fully a father. Finally he came to the conviction that the power to create life was given by God to mankind and, although denied it himself, he could share in it through human solidarity. [10] His wife found herself concerned for a while about who "the other man" would be, and what kind of personality he had.

But ultimately she came to feel very close to her husband, to see the other man as just an agent, and to feel "our" baby would be coming. She anticipated that sharing the pregnancy and birth with him would strengthen his growing feeling that it was their baby.

The Task Force saw that these couples had to work through conflicting, complex needs, feelings and values, and to accept inevitable ambiguities. We saw that they had had to honestly test themselves, their relationship and their future, before reaching a decision which they really wanted to be a responsible one. We do not wish to suggest either that we consider these cases especially well-suited to A.I.D. or that all of us agree with the couples' decision. Had we been involved in counselling them, some of us might have encouraged them to consider whether they might respond to other needs unfolding in their lives, by another kind of choice. But all of us accept the need for contextual decision making. We agree that the choice must be left to the consciences of the individuals who will live out the consequences and to the sense of responsibility of the physician, and that these must make up their minds in a situation without clear-cut black and white answers.

It was against this experiential background that we began to sort out the ethical issues involved in A.I.D.

ETHICAL ISSUES

Background

THE CHURCH OF ENGLAND'S POSITION

Since A.I.D. was studied in depth by a commission appointed by the Archbishop of Canterbury in 1945, we examined the report it issued in 1948, *Artificial human insemination*. The commission received first-hand accounts from doctors giving A.I.D. and it was convinced they were sincerely impelled by compassionate desire to help patients whose sterility often brought great emotional distress and resentment which sometimes put their marriages in jeopardy. It reported some couples had given eloquent testimony to their joy in the new baby, the increased happiness of their marriage, and their gladness both that the wife had found a natural fulfilment for her desires and that they had avoided the risks of adopting a child of unknown parentage. It noted that those who knew them thought that "couples who desire A.I.D. are of more than the average intelligence, thoughtfulness, and responsibility."[11]

Yet, in the end, the commission judged artificial insemination with donated semen to be "wrong in principle and contrary to Christian standards" and it urged that it involved evils so grave that legislation should be framed quickly to make it a criminal offence.[12]

One of the bases of this judgment was a theological understanding of the purposes of sexuality and marriage deduced in part from a physical analysis of sexual organs and functions. (Dissenting member W.R. Matthews, Dean of St. Paul's, considered it a static understanding of human nature and society.) Although it recorded with apparent sympathy the view that A.I.D. was free of the harmful intentions and consequences of adultery, it saw A.I.D. as a wrongful indulgence of a woman's inordinate parental desires which indeed might be based on a rejection of human creatureliness. Emphasizing the intensely personal character of procreation, it saw A.I.D. as "the acme of [the] depersonalization of sex" extracting procreation from human relationships.[13] The giving and receiving of the seed of a man other than her husband was held to be an act of intercourse, so both married woman and donor were committing adultery in A.I.D. Thus it held that A.I.D. violates the exclusive union between husband and wife and involves a breach of the marriage.[14] Another ground for their judgment was their view that physical kinship is the basis of the family upon which moral obligations are erected and these might not survive if that kinship were put in doubt.[15] The commission deplored the fact that fraud and deception were regularly practised on both family and society by the usual registration of the A.I.D. child as a normally conceived child of the marriage, although by the relevant legal definitions it was clearly illegitimate. Such registration unjustly deceived relatives, might defeat their claims to succession and titles and involved a criminal offence. The secrecy on which everyone insisted with regard to A.I.D., the risks connected to disclosure, and the motivation and intentions of the donor raised further serious doubts for them.

Thus moral indignation, founded on theological understandings, joined legal concern and led the commission to condemn A.I.D. severely.

W.R. Matthews, in dissent, asserted that it would be very difficult to prohibit the simple technique of A.I.D. and A.I.D. could be viewed as adulterous "only on a crassly materialistic hypothesis of the meaning of the words."[16] But he expressed fear that in separating the mechanical factor in procreation from the personal, organic life of the individual, A.I.D. might "strike a blow" at the intimate union of body and personality, degrade our conception of personality and ultimately have a disastrous effect on the health of society.[17]

THE FEVERSHAM REPORT

When the British government set up the Feversham committee to study A.I.D. a decade later, the Archbishop of Canterbury upheld the 1948 conclusion. The committee he appointed advised that although A.I.D. should not be made a criminal offence, it should be equated with adultery or fornication (according to circumstances), by legislation, if necessary.[18]

The Feversham report also expressed an adverse judgment on A.I.D. It thought that a wife's receiving of the seed of a person other than her husband "would go against what has hitherto been regarded as the essential nature of marriage,"[19] and that the donor showed a lack of responsibility. In its view A.I.D. was both undesirable and unwise since it carried risks for the relationship between the husband and wife concerned, and also for the child's psychological development. Indeed it was a grave injustice to the intended child, might raise other children's doubts about their true parentage, and was a matter of public concern as it "may well disturb the harmony of society."[20] Although the committee held that A.I.D. should neither be prohibited nor regulated by law, it hoped the practice might diminish or entirely disappear.

A dissenting memorandum was submitted by two members who did not favour encouraging A.I.D. but thought it might be properly employed in a small number of stable marriages. They found it difficult to understand the committee's view that A.I.D. violated the principle of monogamy, and they urged that children born of A.I.D. to which the mother's husband had consented should be registered as his legitimate children.[21]

REPORT OF THE ROYAL COMMISSION ON FAMILY AND CHILDREN'S LAW IN BRITISH COLUMBIA, MAY 1975

Late in our study the report on artificial insemination issued by this B. C. Royal Commission was brought to our attention. In its brief two pages on ethical issues, the commission suggested that in reaching ethical conclusions many would want to hold in tension the opposing responses of confident hope and anxiety which people make to advances in biomedical technology.

Noting that it had considered opposing arguments on the rights of individuals and the common good, and the effects of social policy and legislation, it concluded that "Social policy and legislation concerning AID should not prohibit the procedure, nor should it (sic) promote its use." In its view no individual has an "unfettered right to AID" and thus "guidelines should be laid down to govern AID in order to enable physicians to provide AID in a rational and socially acceptable way."[22]

In the light of these reports the Task Force defined a number of key issues needing ethical reflection and decision.

Marriage and Values

We had to ask first: does A.I.D. fit with our understanding of the nature and purposes of marriage? In what ways? Does it cut across these purposes? Is it a morally acceptable and justifiable procedure for a Christian couple?

ADULTERY

A.I.D. was condemned as adultery and as a breach of the exclusive union of husband and wife by the 1948

Church of England commission. Some of the Task Force felt impatient with the notion that A.I.D. should be regarded as adultery and therefore rejected. To ordinary people adultery occurs when a married person engages in coitus with someone to whom he or she is not married. Since A.I.D. precisely avoids personal intimacy between the man who provides the sperm and the woman who receives it, and is acceptable to many couples for this very reason, the term adultery seems peculiarly misapplied to A.I.D.

Unfaithfulness to a spouse is one essential constituent of adultery, in a Christian perspective. Where a couple openly and mutually choose A.I.D. there is no betrayal of their trust in each other. Nor is there an interruption of their marital fellowship by the kind of personal relationship that marital unfaithfulness usually connotes.

Before insemination techniques were developed, the semen of a man other than her husband could enter a woman's body only by adulterous copulation. It is not surprising, then, that, by reversal of the thought, the presence of such semen, although effected by insemination, was considered to constitute adultery, and the process itself to be analagous to adultery. This kind of interpretation was the more readily made at a point when procreation was regarded as the primary purpose of coitus and the semen was there in order to cause conception. But in A.I.D. we are not dealing with the personal, sexual break in marital union which adultery represents, nor with its hurtful and sinful aspects.

The medical technique of A.I.D. thus seems to us to fail to resemble adultery in significant ways. Considering what we think adultery is and why it is wrong, we would not oppose A.I.D. on grounds that it was adulterous.

But there are reasons why people may continue to think of A.I.D. as adulterous and wrong. Historically, in different cultures and periods, adultery has been defined in other ways and condemned for reasons other than those just mentioned. It is probable the view that adultery is a violation of male property rights in the female lies behind the ten commandments. Adultery has also been abhorred as a violation of the integrity of the male's blood-line. And it has been condemned as a violation of a taboo system devised to enable man to enter and handle the area of sex conceived of as sacred and otherwise dangerously explosive. (Such a taboo system subjected sex, which in primitive minds was both holy and polluted, to rituals of betrothal, marriage, purification and acceptance of the newborn, as well as to taboos governing the persons with whom sexual intercourse is acceptable.) In the opinion of Task Force member Paul Gibson, the classical Christian position on marriage, which stressed the one-flesh unity symbolic of Christ's union with his church, was also partly based on this understanding of sex as a sacred area of human experience, an understanding moreover which Paul's deep suspicion of sex echoed. Gibson suggests that these understandings of adultery are handed on in family lore and folk traditions and "may belong to what Jung called the collective memory of humanity" and he believes "the psychological forces which produced the treatment of sex as sacred are not dead but only suppressed."[23] Thus these understandings may still be of importance in society today. Where people see adultery as a violation of the integrity of the male's blood-line, they will consider A.I.D., which clearly does this, to be adultery. And where people consciously or subconsciously are committed to an atavistic view of sex as sacred and/or polluted, A.I.D. may be felt to be adultery. Thus it may continue to be regarded as adulterous and wrong by some, the more so since A.I.D. is still new to the public and has often been so described by church authorities.

THE MARRIAGE RELATIONSHIP AND PROCREATION

The Task Force thinks that serious reflection on marriage and its purposes is needed in order to arrive at a valid conclusion about A.I.D. Two somewhat different viewpoints were expressed by its members.

The Traditional view

Our understanding of marriage as a one-flesh unity ordained by God is based on the teachings of the New Testament in which the Genesis understanding of marriage was expanded into a high ideal.[24] Man and woman are to join together under God in a mutual love marked by fidelity, exclusiveness and permanence and mirroring in its self-gift and sacrifice the total commitment of Christ to his bride, the church. Marriage of course is to be lived out according to the single great command in which the ten commandments were caught up and expressed afresh: thou shalt love the Lord thy God and thy neighbour as thyself. In the prayerbook wedding service which is based on this understanding, marriage exists for dedicating and sanctifying the union between man and woman, the procreation of children to be christianly brought up, and the mutual society, help and comfort of the two whose lives are joined. The questions asked in this service — wilt thou love him (her), comfort, honour and help him (her), in sickness and in health, and forsaking all other keep thee only unto him (her) so long as you both shall live — and the solemn promises made, make it plain that the pair should undertake marriage in a spirit of unreserved good will. They are to fully join their lives, for all time, come what may. They are to enter married life to serve God together, for their own salvation and his glory.

How should we understand the place of procreation

within such a marriage relationship? In the wedding service, after the questions and promises, prayers are offered asking God to help the pair fulfil their undertakings and to grant them the blessings of married life — perfect love, peace and children.

To some of us, this implies that in the Anglican tradition marriage is, in essence, the joining together of a man and a woman in a mutual life. But everything else — harmony, good health, fortune, children — is a blessing not guaranteed with the marriage; failure and disappointment will be crosses in the providential unfolding of life.

For us, a couple who found that giving themselves to each other in sexual union did not bring the blessing of children, might still live their married life to the glory of God, as the church calls them to do, by dedicating themselves to other kinds of service. For some holding this view, faithful love responsive to the will of God would mean accepting infertility, refusing A.I.D. as being outside the realm of mutual self-giving, and channeling energies in other directions, possibly into responding to the many needs of children and youth in our society.

Critique

Such a traditional view may seem closed to new possibilities which did not exist when the church's ritual was developed. Its shift of emphasis concerning the purposes of marriage does seem to be in line with the way many young people are now approaching marriage.[25]

The argument that childlessness should be accepted as part of the "worse" involved in the marriage commitment is, however, a "broad argument that tends to be better as a pastoral solution to help people when there are no other possibilities," as Roman Catholic moral theologian Charles Curran observed. [26] Some members of the Task Force consider that it subjects persons to biological processes making the biological consequences of fleshly activity sacrosanct and inviolable in a way that is inconsistent with other stances Anglicans have taken. Anglicans do not hold that mutual self-giving in coitus necessitates being bound fully to its biological consequences. We have accepted that couples may limit the full natural effects of coitus by using birth control. Although conception follows more certainly and naturally from coitus than do other natural results which may accompany it, yet we have accepted the couple's right to birth control on the understanding that deepening affection and unity are also important values of coitus. So these may be valid reasons for intervening to prevent the other natural consequence, procreation. Nor do we hesitate to intervene in the natural processes of pregnancy and childbirth with intra-uterine blood transfusions, caesarian section, anaesthesia and incubators to assist when nature does not give the baby its best chance to survive.

In these aspects of marital life we have departed from our ancestors' acceptance of nature as providence. We have already decided it is morally right for us to exercise human freedom and to make choices circumventing the natural processes of coitus in one way, according to humanly chosen values, believing that we can thereby attain the fullness of life that God intends for us. In the traditional natural law understanding of sexuality and marriage, procreation was seen as the final end of genital activity, and this biological finality provided a cohesive sex and marital ethic.[27] But today we see a diversity of human values as natural to sexual activity within marriage, with no one of these as the final end, and we believe persons must responsibly choose amongst them. We no longer read a normative definition of marriage and marital duties from nature but stress personal relationship and fulfilment. If persons may morally use contraception to pursue the human value of deepening conjugal love, without pursuing the natural value of procreation, the question may validly be raised: may they not also morally use A.I.D. to attain the human fulfilment of having children?

In our biblical tradition, the Genesis creation myth celebrates God's gift to man of the power to create life. It tells of God's command to man to be fruitful and multiply, and places a high value on the blessing of children. The Old Testament also records that in the struggle to survive, the Hebrews at times resorted to procreating children outside the marriage bed, as the story of Sarah and Hagar illustrates.[28] While sharing the New Testament's high ideal of marriage and affirming the centrality of love, some members of the Task Force believe that faithful love responsive to the will of God can mean coming to terms with sterility and disappointment, renouncing humiliation and pride, and finding greater service in mutual support in having A.I.D.

How shall we regard A.I.D.?

Implicit in the positive answer some give to the question of the moral acceptability of A.I.D. is the view that A.I.D. is just the introduction by medical technique of a fertilizing agent (the donor's semen) and does not damage the integrity of the couple's marital relationship. Such a view stresses that faithfulness is the essential personal bond between the pair, that parenthood is a moral relationship with children, and that they may attain a more fully human life through meeting their need to bear children.[29] Whether A.I.D. is acceptable, then, would have to be explored individually and contextually within the broad parameters of a given couple's married life, in the light of the fundamental ethical obligation all Christians have to live their lives in love. The tests would be whether it is a truly loving and responsible choice for both, freely, equally and mutually arrived at, and whether either, or others close to them, or their community, are being seriously hurt by it. Values relevant to personal relationships within the specific social context would serve as the criteria for whether A.I.D. was a morally justifiable choice within a given marriage.

Some members of the Task Force, however, question whether the view that A.I.D. is just a technical intervention takes into full account the human dimensions of the experience the couple will go through. The decision to have A.I.D. is a personal choice made on intellectual and emotional grounds and can be shared fully by husband and wife. As a pair they promised to be one and have by the choice of A.I.D. faithfully preserved their personal bodily union. But the realities of the ensuing pregnancy also include the bodily reality that the child the woman bears comes genetically from an unknown father whom it will resemble in looks and personality, to some degree. The processes of pregnancy may well foster her sense of identity with her child or lay a physiological basis for later maternal attachment and care. [30] But it is not unreasonable to suspect the child will have an "otherness" to which she may sometimes feel stranger. It is normal and beautiful for a woman to see and love her husband in the child born of their mutual love. Both wife and husband may later, as parents, be conscious of the anonymity of the genetic father of their A.I.D. child and experience insecurities or conflict about this. Thus some of us think the view that A.I.D. is a technical intervention may not take seriously enough the psychosomatic unity of human personality and the full dimensions of the human experiences involved in childbearing and parenting.[31]

If we think of the donor, A.I.D. involves him in

separating his powers to create new life from personal caring for that life. Does such action go counter to or does it simply cut across the integrated sexual morality evolved in Christian thinking?[32] Some of us believe that donors can participate from a personal conviction that theirs is a responsible act, a humane and generous response to legitimate needs that cannot otherwise be met. Others question whether mature men would find it easy to so detach themselves from the serious consequences of their actions without denial, anxiety or risk of trivializing their sexuality. Connecting bodily activity with moral and social responsibility seems important if we are to be whole, caring persons.

Is there behind the view that A.I.D. is a mechanical intervention a concept that the body can be readily subjected to the will, of body-mind duality which runs counter to Christian understandings of man? "If we are to arrive at any definition of what is good or harmful for man, clearly we must move from some interpretation and evaluation of what man truly is."[33] In short, what is a loving action must be decided by looking at what man is. It seems important to reflect on the biblical affirmation that man is made in the image of God in a personhood in which body and soul are one entity.[34]

Some of us have doubts that the concept of A.I.D. as a technical intervention rests on a holistic understanding of man and suspect it involves some denial of realities. So for us there remains a question whether A.I.D. is supportive or destructive of authentic human purposes and relationships. Although we are concerned, we do not have any simple or final answers. Carefully researched evidence of how A.I.D. affects persons and their relationships would help us to know whether it should be regarded as a procedure truly fulfilling human purposes. But the practice of secrecy has meant that only a small number of limited reports by the practitioners themselves have been published.

We would be more persuaded that A.I.D. could indeed be fully integrated as a human experience if the couples and medical personnel involved could be wholly honest about the realities of what A.I.D. is, honest with themselves, with others, including the child if the need arose, and with the community. Openness and honesty would argue that conflicts have been resolved and that the experience does not split will and deeds from feelings. The present insistence that A.I.D. is merely a technical intervention and the practice of secrecy leave room for doubt about whether those involved can fully accept the realities of A.I.D.

The family

Would A.I.D. foster or work against the kind of family Christians want to establish? First, we think that families both are and should be based on moral bonds of caring and trust. A husband and wife's acceptance of responsibility for children, mutual consent to belong in a family and solidarity are the actual bases and strengths of families in our divorce-prone society. Although some of us, in the light of our understanding of human nature and marriage, have reservations about the acceptability of A.I.D., we do not share the view expressed in the Church of England's 1948 report that physical kinship is the inescapable foundation of family and its bond.

Some of us are concerned about the effect upon the family of the present practice of secrecy concerning A.I.D. Deliberate concealing of significant facts within a family seems to us a serious and questionable step. When we have answered the question of whether A.I.D. is morally acceptable to us, we will discuss this issue more fully later on in this report. The present practice is certainly an understandable one. While there is uncertainty about how others will react to the knowledge that a couple had used A.I.D. and about how far it is really acceptable in our society, there may be reason for couples to fear that telling a child the truth about its A.I.D. origins might be destructive and thus to keep the matter secret. Nevertheless, whether secrecy is really needed to make a success of the procedure or the parenthood is open to question. In any case for some of us there seems to be "real weight" to the objection that "A.I.D. weakens family ties by its secrecy and deception."[35]

We have little information about how family relationships develop where A.I.D. has created the child. There are scattered indications in the literature and in court records of the unhappy results of A.I.D. in some families. The small number of such reports, however, tends to make the practitioners' claim that A.I.D. creates happy families seem reasonable. Certainly families created in the normal way are involved in the large number of marital breakdowns and divorces in our society. Only research of the kind not now available could confirm that A.I.D. creates happy families with little risk of serious hurt to family members. Data would help us to know whether, as some psychologists have suggested, it is harder for the husband who chooses A.I.D. to really involve himself in the later care of the child so conceived, and whether there are risks he will feel doubt about his adequacy as a male or withdraw into occupational concerns.[36] Again, it would be helpful to know if A.I.D. mothers run a risk of becoming overprotective towards the child, or experience conflicts or serious tension in their marital relationship related to their use of donor insemination. We would like to know more about the real effects of A.I.D. upon relationships in the family it creates.

Traditional values and the challenge of the new

Our study brought us sharply up against painful conflicts between deeply held traditional values and powerful new hopes. The belief that "a child is brought into being because two people want their union to be incarnated" led one of us to conclude that were he in need of A.I.D., allowing another man loved by both of them to create a child with his wife through mutual personal love would be more human and would fit his values better. Somehow the use of technical means took the "heart" out of this intensely meaningful human experience for him. Yet his wife thought that the emotional involvement of coitus — in itself clearly adulterous — would make resort to the impersonal technique of insemination necessary in order to safeguard the marriage bond. Another felt that his image of himself as a successful male would be too threatened by A.I.D., that he personally was not strong enough to accept a donor replacing him in the role of progenitor. And he thought the felt pressures of women's liberation might make others cling to this traditional image and value. One of us felt strongly that for her A.I.D. would be a radical turning away from her husband, and the child would bring painful awareness of its "faceless" father and inner conflict damaging her sense of wholeness. Then again another felt it was rationally and morally wrong to separate deliberately producing sperm to cause conception from taking personal responsibility for the life created, that it was contrary to the moral understandings the church had led him to.

But we had to recognize that these values were matched by other values equally derived from our faith. One of us stressed that for Christians children are a blessing and gift and that this understanding derives from God's command to man, recorded in the bible, to be fruitful and multiply and, as well, from the felt desire most human beings experience to continue their own life in children. The value of the *bonum prolis* has to be balanced with the value of personal unity imaged in the one-flesh ideal of marriage. While A.I.D. might entail some revision of traditional concepts of marriage, the church is sensitive to the reality that childless marriages can become self-centred. In this connection preventing the relationship from growing might itself be sinful. The church has always recognized that the responsibility for creating and caring for new life belongs to married couples and might deepen their relationship and bring them into a wider circle of concern. It has valued procreation as a social good — the contribution of the married to society — and a personal good in developing the couple and their relationship.

On the other hand, some of us consider that the moral validity of A.I.D. must be seen in the context of the realities that our world is already overpopulated and that we are confronted with serious world-wide problems of social injustice, resource depletion, pollution and poverty. In the light of the emerging and urgent needs to which we must respond, we wonder if the church has a responsibility to refrain from building social pressures on couples to have children. At this point in history women are also, for the first time, being encouraged to discover an independent identity of their own and the view that woman's fulfilment lies in maternity is rightly being both questioned and regarded as a damaging stereotype. Perhaps the church should assist couples to come to terms creatively with their situation in a variety of different ways, rather than emphasizing children as a supreme good of marriage.

It is clear from our ethical discussion thus far that our understandings of Christian teachings and values cut both ways—they pull some of us towards and some of us away from A.I.D. We think that when decisions are being made about using technological means having a deep impact on persons and on their marriage, it is important that Christians wrestle with the values made known in scripture and in the church's tradition, and with what the commandments recreated in Christ's law of love imply about marital partnership, fidelity, self-sacrifice, and the purposes and limits of human freedom.

We are deeply aware of the need and anguish felt by childless couples. We also felt the pull of the challenge that two joined as one could seek A.I.D. in real mutuality and of the promise that parenthood would enrich their lives through their generous self-giving. We know that all our choices are imperfect and that we must live with ambiguity, not resting content with present structures but pressing on to greater fullness of life through the growth and change which God makes possible and through which he lovingly sustains us. We know we have to confront conflicting pulls and make choices without certainty, accepting ambiguity as part of life.

Technology and freedom

In a wider sense, the tension and ambiguity which we experienced in exploring these moral issues stem from the reality that man has been created free but also, in changing ways, limited, as a creature within the created given world. He lives in an inescapable contradiction between freedom and necessity, and his technological powers painfully confront him with the responsibility of redefining these. A.I.D. presents the basic dilemma of technology: what ought we to use our ever-increasing powers to do, and what are the limits which we ought to place on our freedom?

The matching terms of the freedom-nature equation are not easy to establish. On the one hand, in the biblical perspective of creation, "man as the image of God transcends nature."[37] The Genesis creation myth records that he has been commanded and given the power to have dominion over the natural world. Thus intervention in nature is part of his very nature; in Christian understanding, human, rational and personal transcendence over the material and biological is written into creation itself. Man is also called to grasp his own reality and unfold the possibilities that lie in it. And in a real sense man's creative advance towards seeking ends by choice, controlling and transcending natural restrictions as they relate to his own person can be a human and spiritual victory.[38]

But in using his creativity and freedom man must also confront the question of his own creaturehood. In making his choices, he must take seriously his own finitude under God and the reality that he must answer to God for the use he makes of his powers.

The command to have dominion over the world has been interpreted since the Renaissance, and indeed until recently, as a sanction to completely subdue nature to himself. But today, in a renewed and humbler perspective, theologians, social scientists and scientists are urging that man's vocation is rather to shape the earth, fostering a harmony with the natural world in which earth's plants and animals will be preserved and man's true humanity can grow.[39]

Amongst the diverse possibilities for his self-development, for which God makes him responsible, he must choose those which serve the good of the human person, which enhance his wholeness and dignity, which make him and his life more fully human, for these alone will bring him the development which proceeds from God.[40] When choosing the courses he will pursue, man must always remain aware and test the possibility that tampering with bodily structures and processes may bring risks of serious damage to human personality and personal relationships.

"Neither biblical faith nor the modern sciences of man encourage us to treat the body as a mere object, to be manipulated by some detached mind; on the contrary, for both the unity of human personality and human bodiliness is a primary conviction."[41]

And therein lies the dilemma. For taking seriously that "man is not merely his freedom but also his corporality"[42] means asking whether linking the personal experience of sexual union with begetting and parenthood is an important part of man's humanity. Will the first step severing this link — A.I.D.—turn out to be part of a dehumanizing process?[43] In the 1970s we are only too keenly aware that through technology we have despoiled our planet. We no longer have an optimistic and unlimited faith in science. Nor are we willing to accept the inevitability of technology implied in yesterday's maxim: "If it can be done, it will be done." People are searching man's moral heritage afresh for the truly human criteria by which choices can be made, and they are clear that "no" is sometimes the right answer to technological possibilities.

On the other hand, it is surely factually true that we have already removed the procreative dimension from most sexual union, through birth control. It may also cogently be argued that sexual love is sometimes itself dehumanizing since it is used in lust, selfishness and hatred.[44] Human sexuality must be recognized to be an ambiguous moral basis for creating children when many women in our society who become pregnant through natural means either seek abortion, or, especially in the case of the very young, in worrying numbers do not even know for certain who has fathered their child.[45] Indeed the numbers of children conceived by natural means outside the marital bond far exceed the numbers likely to be produced by A.I.D., so reasonableness and a sense of proportion are very much needed if one is to arrive at a sound judgment on A.I.D. The mature couple who decide on A.I.D. may indeed seem to be pursuing human values in a more responsible way than many other couples procreating naturally.

We have struggled to understand what expresses and realizes the best in human nature, what will make life more fully human. We know we must accept that "we are God's creation under the forms of evolution,"[46] that God is involved in ongoing creation and change is rooted in the very being of things. So our understanding of God and man must embrace change. John Macquarrie surely speaks for many Christians when he affirms that "man really *is* . . . when he ventures forward in hope."[47] We know that Christians ought to look to the future with dynamic hope, in faith that God is with us, helping us to grow as persons through renewing and redemptive change.

While our theological consideration of the dilemma posed by human nature and technology gives no definitive answers, it raises questions which those making choices should wrestle with and suggests tests by which to evaluate experience.

Ethical stance

Thus we believe that A.I.D. confronts us with multiple conflicting values. We think there are no clear-cut easy answers. We have not found any moral absolute that necessitates our rejecting A.I.D. On the other hand, A.I.D. is by no means free of moral ambiguities. If we refuse to accept A.I.D. do we risk absolutizing natural processes and normal relationships? By limiting freedom do we disappoint God-given hopes of creating new life? As Christians healed through God's love in Jesus Christ, we ourselves are called to help redeem the brokenness of our world. Is this a case to which we should respond positively in faith and love? We are certainly called to shape the change built into our world and our nature with generosity of imagination and heart and with belief in God's presence to keep us in his ways as we conscientiously seek to know what he is showing us through our experience.

While some of us still have doubts and questions about A.I.D., most of us believe it is a morally acceptable procedure for doctors to undertake and for some couples to choose. We know that human life is uniquely precious to God who creates and redeems it, and that we must not procreate irresponsibly. So we think a couple should take care to reach a conscientious responsible decision. We believe they should test their choice seriously, honestly considering the values and principles involved and the circumstances of their marriage, their lives and A.I.D. itself. We believe they ought to consider a wide context when making their choice. We would hope the couple would reach a decision which they can wholly enter into, with integrity of body and mind, one which will lead to authentic fulfilment in their lives. We would hope donors would participate from a personal conviction that semen donation is a responsible act.

We turn now to consider the current practice of A.I.D. in specific detail.

MEDICAL ASPECTS

For the physician involved in providing A.I.D. as a medical service, major concerns are: the selection of semen donors, the selection of couples for A.I.D., and the best methods of working with them.

Donors

Dr. Kerr suggested to the Task Force that the selection of donors is not a major problem. Donors are recruited and chosen on the basis of willingness, absence of known illness (especially venereal diseases) or heritable undesirable traits, and acceptable quality of seminal fluid. They are also usually paid for the donation.[48] Physicians often recruit medical students although some prefer married donors who have produced children.[49] J.H. Edwards, professor of human genetics at Birmingham Maternity Hospital, told a CIBA symposium on A.I.D. and embryo transfer in 1972 that "from the technical aspect a genetic expert would have no particular advantage over an intelligent general practitioner in choosing a suitable donor." And as Lord Kilbrandon, British legal authority, then observed, "most of us when we get married take our chances on genetic history."[50]

Yet some authorities are calling for a higher degree of care. In his book *The public policy dimensions of artificial insemination and human-semen cryobanking*, M.S. Frankel has urged that we need stringent medical and genetic tests of donors, since the potential economic and social costs extend beyond the individual donor and recipient. He notes that while most recessive genetic diseases cannot now be detected through screening tests, at least 60 can. Thus society may have to resolve cost-benefit problems taking certain steps to maximize the safety and well-being of recipients and their potential offspring.[51] In its May 1975 report, the British Columbia Royal Commission, drawing on the expertise of geneticists in its working group, recommended that the physician take a carefully detailed family history, conduct a physical examination, and undertake chromosome studies and metabolic studies as prescribed by genetic consultants, in order to detect deleterious dominant genes and chromosome aberrations.[52] It noted that the Rhesus factor should also be recorded so that an Rh negative mother with an Rh problem is not given semen from an Rh positive donor likely to cause haemolytic disease of the newborn. In its view the donor's physical characteristics should also be compatible with those of the recipients, and blood characteristics be compatible with paternity by the child's presumed father, to protect against unintended exposure of the child's origin. The commission further recommended that the donor should be given a psychological evaluation which should include a consideration of the effects that his involvement might have on his wife and household, and that counselling should be provided both to screen out the individual who might be psychologically stressed and to prepare him and his relatives for any stresses arising from "the special future relationships that will never be identified."[53]

As the practice of A.I.D. develops the professionals involved may well be required to extend and deepen the care given in relation to the donor.

The medical technique of insemination

The time of ovulation of the recipient is assessed by an accurate menstrual record. Since menstrual cycles are often irregular, exact prediction is seldom possible and more commonly only a period of 3 or 4 days can be identified. A number of techniques can be used to try to pin-point the time[54] and drugs can sometimes be employed to control the timing of ovulation. However generally insemination has to be performed on two or more occasions in each cycle at a time determined by its length and regularity. The procedure itself takes about 20 minutes and is a simple one, equivalent to a "Pap smear". Fresh seminal fluid is deposited in the cervical canal or upper vagina around the cervix. On average, it takes three or four cycles for conception to occur but it can take very much longer. The success rate depends on the selection of patients but may be as high as 75%.[55] Although the technique is simple, donor insemination is usually stressful and time consuming. Dr. Kerr regards it as "a tedious, inconvenient, repetitive procedure, punctuated by disappointments, but ultimately successful in a reasonable number of couples."[56] It is evident that donor insemination requires the use of both considerable professional skills and medical facilities, and that there is therefore a substantial cost in this service, met of course normally by health insurance.

Recipients

Correct selection of recipients is the major medical problem in Dr. Kerr's opinion. "Relatively little has been written to clarify this area. Criteria for selection have not been clearly identified and there is no consensus of opinion regarding the most appropriate methods of selection."[57] Nor have there been any long-term comprehensive follow-up studies which could provide scientific data about how to select couples for whom A.I.D. will be an enriching and positive experience.

The physician's problem is to select from the couples who satisfy the physical medical criteria those who would be appropriate recipients of A.I.D.

MEDICAL CRITERIA

The husband

Donor insemination is appropriate where investigation establishes that the husband produces no sperm and is sterile, or has consistently low sperm counts in semen specimens and is significantly subfertile.[58] Less commonly, he may be fertile but be the carrier of a dominant heritable illness such as Huntington's chorea, or of cystic fibrosis, or he may be Rh positive with an Rh negative wife who has had a pregnancy complicated by Rh immunization. His infertility may be associated with a general illness jeopardizing his health and life, but this may not constitute an absolute bar.[59] In Dr. Kerr's opinion "where the man's life is currently threatened . . . any decision regarding donor insemination should be delayed until the crisis is resolved;" even where the husband is incapacitated or his long-term future is uncertain, the couple might qualify for A.I.D. provided they have discussed and clearly understand the situation.[60]

The wife

Thorough investigation, with use of laparoscopy, dye transit and endometrial biopsy, should establish that she has no impairment to conception. The physician should also establish that her health will not compromise the outcome of pregnancy and that her life expectancy is reasonable. Where difficulties related to pelvic disorders are found, treatment may make insemination possible. Severe diabetes might be a contraindication and Dr. Kerr stated that "one would be guarded in accepting a woman over 37."

PSYCHOLOGICAL CRITERIA

It is essential that both husband and wife have come to terms with their infertility and with the many painful feelings they will inevitably have about it. The man "should not feel his masculinity [is] threatened. He must be tolerant of the idea of not being the biological father of his child, and have an appreciation that it is in the social role of fatherhood that fulfilment lies rather than in the biological role."[61] The woman "should have accepted the fact of her husband's inability to inseminate her successfully and have been able to express and deal with her consequent feelings. The wife must not be using a demand for donor insemination as revenge for her husband's failure to give her a child."[61]

Dr. Kerr said he "would at present consider only married heterosexual unions, and would not consider either single women or lesbian couples as prospective parents."

It is important that the couple discuss their feelings and reach a common ground of agreement. They must also resolve moral or religious doubts and be sure about their commitment. Dr. Kerr insists "the couple must have a stable, mature relationship," and "must be seen to communicate freely and honestly with each other." Their motivation for children "should be based on a mature judgement, and not simply be a response to peer or parental pressures. A pregnancy should certainly not be sought as a means of holding together an unstable marriage. Both members of the couple should share the desire for a child. . . . They should not be overly concerned about donor selection. If the child *must* have certain specific physical characteristics or mental capabilities, then this couple may have not fully come to grips with donor insemination." And lastly, "a sense of complete trust must be present between the couple and the [medical] team."

The physician's role

Dr. Kerr considers the criteria for selecting recipients are "ill-defined and subjective, [and] they are difficult to apply in the clinical situation." He thinks the physician can benefit by the support of a team and in his practice a female nurse practitioner shared in infertility interviews. Current women's literature claims that the medical system has been "a prime source of sexist ideology and an enforcer of sex roles"[62] and that male doctors still display insensitive, authoritarian attitudes towards women. Thus a male-female professional team would seem highly appropriate for this kind of service where real sensitivity is needed.

Where donor insemination is relevant joint involvement of husband and wife is essential, so individual interviews should be complemented by interviews involving the couple. There is real advantage in having a male-female professional team to elucidate and assess the couple's feelings and motivation, and the strengths and weaknesses of their marital relationship. Dr. Kerr is very opposed to decisions being hastily arrived at in a single visit, and notes "there may be a tendency for the interviewers to feel under pressure, but this has to be resisted." He emphasizes the positive value in insisting on a few months delay between the interview and taking the decision, to allow time for reconsideration, and he has found that many couples later confirmed this waiting time was of value.

Dr. Kerr thinks the infertility team should have consultant support. While a physician may feel he is best equipped to make decisions concerning his patients and may resent delegating responsibility, nevertheless a consultant group including a psychiatrist and social worker experienced in problems of human reproduction, and possibly a clergyman and a lawyer with insight into moral and legal questions might provide valuable assistance.[63] Problem patients might be referred to such a group (assuming the fertility team can recognize these), or, alternatively, the group could participate in all decisions about donor insemination. Collectively they might more accurately predict a couple's ability to handle donor insemination, offer expert resources and observe their patients over an adequate period of time to assess the validity of their judgments.

The physician himself must fully inform the couple about all aspects of A.I.D., including the practical logistics, chances of success or failure, legal implications, and the fact that the wife has no greater but no less risk of having a miscarriage or an abnormal child than any other pregnant woman. For his own protection he will need to secure their signatures to a carefully drawn consent form indicating their acceptance of these realities.

Dr. Kerr believes that, when pregnancy is successfully initiated, the physician can play a constructive role by using a family-centred approach to maternity care. He can help the husband to identify with his wife's pregnancy and the coming child by encouraging him to share in training for childbirth and permitting him to be with his wife when she is giving birth. By assisting them to share the whole experience from beginning to end, he can help them to build their relationship as parents on a solid and equal emotional basis. Family-centred maternity care is of particular value to A.I.D. couples, in his opinion.

Ethical issues arising from the medical practice of A.I.D.

RESPONSIBILITY AND THE PHYSICIAN

It seems clear that a physician who wants to choose couples for A.I.D. in a responsible way will need to be able to observe and to understand people's feelings and abilities. It is not easy to discover whether a couple equally and mutually desire A.I.D. Nor is it easy to determine whether they have both a realistic understanding of possible difficulties in their relationships with each other and with their future child, and ability to cope with these. It seems that if they would use A.I.D. responsibly, those giving it must help a couple to open up and must test "where they are at" as persons and as a couple.

Experts with experience in adoption agree with A.I.D. practitioners that the couple's resolution of conflicts about sterility and acceptance that they will have a different kind of parenthood are important. But they add that the success or failure of a family established when couples are sterile depends on the parents' capacity to give warmth and affection to a child. They also emphasize the need to focus on the child and his future needs.[64]

Since medical education is designed to develop competence in medicine, it seems reasonable to anticipate physicians would have skills in evaluating a couples' physical suitability for A.I.D. and in performing the procedure. Medical school does not usually, however, give solid training in understanding interaction within marriage and family, or in counselling. Experience in practice may give a physician considerable working knowledge of human nature. Yet support from those whose skills lie in the field of human relations, marriage and family, and counselling, would seem really important, the more so since the schedules of busy practitioners do not conduce to the investment of substantial time in counselling. With these needs in mind it has even been suggested that an agency such as the Children's Aid Society, with expertise in assessing parental competence and long experience with the related problem of adoption, might logically assume a role in couple selection and counselling, but this seems an extreme solution to us. We see value in the concept of a clinic team in which the physician has an integral role. Wider discussion in seminars and study groups, in which personnel involved in A.I.D. could share with those involved in adoption services, might be of benefit. As well, improved training in medical school or post-graduate professional development could help physicians acquire skills in these areas.

THE DONOR

Several questions seem to need consideration concerning semen donation. The donor is paid apparently in order to secure enough seminal fluid to ensure the care of patients. The principle that persons cannot sell parts of their bodies is widely accepted and seems both wise and just. The sale of human tissues is statutorily forbidden in several jurisdictions (notably Ontario and B.C.) and while blood may be sold, throughout Canada a voluntary system of blood donation has been established to good purpose. If we examine the system of paid blood donation permitted in the U.S. we discover that payment of donors vastly increases the risk of transmission of hepatitis in transfusion, and the infected blood tends to come from alcoholics, drug addicts and prisoners.[65] R.M. Titmuss, author of an important book on the subject, adds the serious charge that "paid donors — and especially poor donors badly in need of money — are . . . less likely to reveal a full medical history."[66] There may be no true parallel between blood donation and semen donation but it is not unreasonable to be uneasy about the kind of person who might want to earn money from semen donation, particularly to large, impersonal semen banks, and to be concerned about the circumstances which might motivate them.[67] It has to be remembered that semen donation can be made much more frequently than blood donation. Might not the irresponsible find this an easy way to earn money, or might not semen be given too frequently by the same person if semen donation is an unregulated private business? Should we regard semen donation as a commercial transaction or is it important that it be a "gift of giving," a service? The latter concept seems to underly the B.C. Royal Commission's suggestion that payment should be in compensation for the donor's loss of time or of revenues due to this loss, and for his expenses.[68] One feels uneasy on learning from one of those involved in A.I.D. practice that "people are not ready at the moment to give their semen free, as we donate blood. Possibly in another 10-20 years people will feel that they are helping couples who cannot have babies."[69]

Most of the Task Force would prefer that the individual physician keep control of semen donation, personally selecting the donor; this seems to provide a better guarantee of careful selection, and to avoid possible errors in labelling to which a semen bank might also be subject. There also seems merit in the B.C. Royal Commission's recommendation that a limit should be placed on the numbers of successful sperm donation that may be provided by any individual donor, since there is a slight risk that abnormalities not detected in donor screening might show up in the children conceived.[70] In view of the possibility of abnormalities, and the additional slight risk that the donor might later develop a heritable disease of genetic origin which might make genetic counselling of the A.I.D. child advisable, it seems obvious that the doctor should keep complete medical records about all semen donations and inseminations.

One further important matter is the nature of the consent form which should be obtained from the donor. In current practice the donor's name is never revealed to the recipient and it is held necessary that the donor never seek to know the names of any recipient or the results of his donations. He must fully accept this anonymity and understand that his donation entails none of the duties or rights of a father towards a child his donation creates. The consent form suggested by the B.C. Royal Commission spells this out in detail and includes a statement that the donor takes full responsibility both for informing his own relatives and for any effects his donation may have on them.[71] The donor should also be aware that his anonymity might be at risk, in the event, for instance, that a defective child was born as a result of the insemination and that litigation concerning the physician's liability ensued. This is a matter to which we will return in the legal section of the report.

SECRECY

Coupled with the assumption that the donor must be anonymous — an assumption which seems psychologically, socially and legally inescapable — is the further assumption accepted by most authorities that the child's A.I.D. origin ought never to be revealed to him. Indeed the B.C. Royal Commission holds compatibility of donor's and parents' physical characteristics important because "the child should not have the fact of his origin by artificial insemination divulged to him."[72] This stance implies that it is both possible and right to maintain secrecy about the matter in front of the child.

But the assumptions that secrecy is possible and that it is right may both be open to serious question. There is certainly some risk that in later marital quarrels one of the partners may unintentionally reveal that the child is *hers* in a deeper sense than it is his.[73] Or that during the normal quarrels with their parents which adolescents have as they struggle towards independence, the adolescent may discover the secret of his origins.[74] In addition to the risk of suspicion or accidental disclosure, legal proceedings concerning divorce, support and adoption have occasionally revealed the circumstances of conception. It is thus at least arguable that secrecy may not be in the child's best interests, in the long run.

In the past, secrecy was the practice in adoption. It may be useful to consider the reasons why adoption authorities now insist the child be told the truth about his adoption. Their insistence "is not based upon any belief that this is an easy thing to do or that the child will have no problems with the truth about himself;" rather it stems from "the conviction that the atmosphere created by secrecy and untruth is even harder to bear and carries the potential for even more serious problems. . . . Denial and concealment consume a great deal of emotional energy which could be better expended in facing and resolving problems. . . . "[75]

Adoption is clearly more difficult to conceal than is conception by A.I.D., so the parallel is not exact. Perhaps it depends on what kind of a secret we are talking about. Whether concealment is possible or right for the married couple may depend on whether artificial insemination is an "emotionally charged" secret which they must deliberately suppress and which will continue to affect them[76] or whether, as many practitioners seem to hold, the insemination is a technical procedure which they quickly forget in the shared anticipation of the child's coming. Interestingly, R.T. Francoeur, a former Catholic priest who has written numerous books enthusiastically supporting the new reproductive techniques, noted both that most A.I.D. couples find it next to impossible to explain their decision to their child, families and friends, and that "psychologically and emotionally, even the more educated . . . find it difficult to cope with the reality and implications of artificial insemination."[77]

Some members of the Task Force feel uneasy about the rightness of any moral action which *must* be kept secret — it goes against our sense of moral integrity. Anything that must be kept secret may have aspects which the persons concerned don't want to face, would rather evade or deny. A sense of personal integrity might rather demand that a man not pretend to himself or to others that he is the biological father and might suggest that fully accepting his child means being fully honest. Yet it must be acknowledged that truth telling may be chosen for destructive motives and be needlessly damaging and there may be serious reasons for not adhering to it in this matter; and this also relates to personal integrity. It may be that telling the child of his origins is not possible because of the present status of illegitimacy of A.I.D. children.[78] Or it may carry risks to preserving the anonymity of the donor. Although in general it might be thought that the confidentiality of medical records provides adequate guarantee of this, in litigation in Canada, at the present time, there is in fact no legally protected right of the patient to have medical records withheld. More open acceptance of A.I.D. in society, together with legal clarification so that the donor is acknowledged to have none of the obligations of fatherhood towards the child and the consenting husband of the inseminated woman is clearly defined as the lawful father of the child might make secrecy unnecessary.[79]

Not all those personally involved in the study or experience of A.I.D. believe secrecy is desirable. British geneticist Anne McLaren told the 1972 CIBA Symposium "probably A.I.D. children should be told of their origins."[78]

American writer Lillian Atallah, herself a mother,

recently revealed in the *New York Times* in articles republished by the *Globe and Mail* that when she was told at 20 of her A.I.D. origins, finding out had been a good experience, giving her a new perspective. Although her parents were warned by their obstetrician that discovery of the secret might give her an irreparable inferiority complex and lead to social maladjustment, she says, "Knowing about my A.I.D. birth did nothing to deplete my feelings for my family. I felt grateful, especially to my father for all the trouble they had taken to give me life."[80] The issue may have been clouded by conjecture which experience and reality might disprove. Atallah considers "the news of a donor-father might well be traumatic to a young child,"[80] so perhaps how and when to tell a child is what we should be thinking about. One of the women seeking A.I.D. whom CTV's W5 interviewed in June 1976 and one of the couples we interviewed thought they would like eventually to tell their child. Certainly leadership and courage will have to come from those personally involved. At least one physician who had always held that telling the child was unnecessary and unwise psychologically, has changed his mind and suggested "we should take a new look in appropriate families" to discover accurately and scientifically what the effects actually are.[81] Perhaps we should be thinking more creatively in terms of privacy and of protecting the respective rights of the couple and the families of both recipient and donor, rather than of secrecy.

THE CHILD'S IDENTITY

We must remember also that the issue of the child's identity is inextricably tied into that of secrecy. And one of the things we have learned in recent years is just how crucial certainty about their biological roots can be for some people whose sense of identity seems to hang on it. The Church of England's 1948 report seems to have made a valid point in holding that "doubt or ignorance as to one's parentage can give rise to acute distress."[82] The search of adopted children for their biological parents is a growing phenomenon today. In Canada, members of Parent Finders, an organization with 300 members which was founded several years ago, told CTV's W5, 13 June 1976, that genetic heritage is important and that the intensive search which they assist is based on a need for continuity of family. Adopted persons recently made strong pleas to a committee of the Ontario Ministry of Community and Social Services appointed to make recommendations on adoption legislation that information about biological parentage should be made available to them; their pleas were moving testimony to the loneliness which they felt originated in their lack of background knowledge.[83] Since the right of adopted children to such information is under legislative study in a number of countries and has already been enacted in Great Britain[84] it may be important for A.I.D. practitioners to consider the implications of this trend.[85]

THE FAMILY

Few studies have been undertaken of the happiness or problems of A.I.D. families and there is no long range study reported in the scientific literature. Atallah mentions a 1955 study of 300 A.I.D. families in which Dr. Alan Guttmacher found "there had been no divorces, the children were well-loved by both parents and there was a general feeling of gratitude for a family made complete."[86] There are a small number of similarly positive reports.[87] Dr. Wayne Decker of the New York Fertility Research Foundation probably speaks for many A.I.D. practitioners when he says that "casual observations would indicate that the feedback from AID is 99 per cent positive."[88] Since there is much more A.I.D. now than just a few years ago, more extended follow-up studies could usefully be undertaken in order to confirm selection criteria and discover problems that might be avoided or ways of dealing with them. When it recommended that A.I.D. be made more widely available through centres set up within the National Health Service, the British Medical Association's Peel Panel (1973) also advised "there should be properly conducted long-term follow-up of these families though it appreciates that there will be difficulties in instituting methods of follow-up which are effective and acceptable."[89] In its view, "information must be obtained on the genetic effects, especially where frozen semen has been used, and it is important to learn the effects, in human terms, on the development of personal relationships in families resulting from the use of AID." The panel's recommendation seems to us to be a reasonable one, to ensure that A.I.D. is done in the best possible way.

LEGAL CONCERNS

Dr. Kerr probably spoke for medical practitioners in general when he represented to the Task Force that the legal position concerning A.I.D. is unclear and should be clarified. In fact there are no legislative enactments in Canada dealing with A.I.D. and the courts here, in England, and in the U.S. have dealt with few cases and have established few if any binding precedents.[90] What legal difficulties might A.I.D. pose, then, for each of the parties involved?

The recipient couple, adultery and divorce

There seems to be some legal uncertainty still as to whether A.I.D. constitutes adultery on the part of the wife receiving it. Turning to judicial decisions, the most famous early case involving A.I.D. was *Orford v. Orford*, decided by the Supreme Court of Ontario in 1921. In the proceedings, in which a wife was suing for alimony, she gave evidence that a child of which her husband was not the father was born to her as a result of artificial insemination undertaken without her husband's consent. Orde J. found as a fact that she had committed adultery in the ordinary way. But then, dealing with the issue of A.I.D. which she had raised, he stated:

> the essence of the offence of adultery consists not in the moral turpitude of the act of sexual intercourse, but in the voluntary surrender to another person of the reproductive powers or faculties of the guilty person; and any submission of those powers to the service or enjoyment of any person other than the husband or the wife comes within the definition of 'adultery'.[91]

This view that A.I.D. is adultery was followed in a 1954

action for divorce in Illinois, *Doornbos v. Doornbos*. However both cases, as Dean G.P.R. Tallin pointed out in a well known article in the *Canadian Bar Review* in 1956 were decided on other grounds and the opinions on A.I.D. were *obiter dicta*.[92]

A more recent and significant judgment was made in *Maclennan v. Maclennan*, 1958, a divorce action on the ground of adultery against a woman who had had A.I.D. without her husband's consent. Here the Scottish Court held that: for adultery to be committed there must be two persons physically present and engaging in the sexual act, with some degree of penetration of the female organ by the male organ, but not necessarily any deposit of male seed in the female's ovum; "the placing of the male seed in the female ovum need not necessarily result from the sexual act and if it does not, but is placed there by some other means, there is no sexual intercourse." In sum, "the extraction of the nexus of human relationship from the act of procreation remove[s] artificial insemination from the classification of sexual intercourse," and hence of adultery.[93] This decision is generally accepted as good law in England.[94] There have been a few English cases in which sexual misconduct falling short of penetration has been held to constitute adultery for purposes of divorce.[95] A reasonable explanation for these conclusions in case law is that they resulted from the pressure on reason and credulity created by rigid divorce laws.[96]

It should be noted that "there is no legal requirement that if the woman is married her husband should consent" to her having A.I.D.[97] A husband's previous written consent to A.I.D. would not alter the nature of the act if in fact a court held A.I.D. to be adulterous, but it would amount to connivance or condonation and form a possible bar to divorce proceedings on his part. Because of the broadening of divorce laws in recent years, however, "the question of whether A.I.D. constitutes adultery may be of less importance as other grounds for divorce now exist. It may be argued in certain circumstances that A.I.D. with or without the husband's consent constitutes "cruelty" of such a kind to be a ground for dissolution of marriage under the *Divorce Act* 1969."[98] In this connection, Lord Wheatley in *Maclennan v. Maclennan* had observed as "almost trite" that a married woman who had artificial insemination by donor without her husband's consent "has committed a grave and heinous breach of the contract of marriage."[99]

B.M. Dickens, formerly of the College of Law, London, England, and now professor at the University of Toronto Law School, considers the judgment in *Maclennan v. Maclennan* that A.I.D. does not constitute adultery in divorce law even when the husband does not consent is notable.[100] Toronto lawyer Rosalie Abella, now a Family Court judge, suggested on CTV's W5, 20 June 1976, that the opinion generally held in legal circles is that A.I.D. would not now be held, in a Canadian court, to be adultery.[101]

Legitimacy of the child

A more thorny question is whether the A.I.D. child is illegitimate. In common law a child begotten through a father who is not the mother's husband is illegitimate; hence a child of a married woman which is conceived and born during the marriage but of which her husband is not the father is illegitimate.

There have been a number of American cases with findings as to the legitimacy of an A.I.D. child. A New York court touched on the question in *Strnad v. Strnad* (1948).[102] In this suit the wife, amongst other claims, sought custody of her child, born of A.I.D. with her husband's consent. The parties agreed the child was not of his blood but in judgment the court held:

> the child has been potentially adopted or semi-adopted by the defendant . . . In the opinion of this Court, assuming again that the plaintiff was artificially inseminated with the consent of the defendant, this child is not an illegitimate child. Indeed, logically and realistically, the situation is no different than that pertaining in the case of a child born out of wedlock who by law is made legitimate upon the marriage of the interested parties.[103]

Dean Tallin has argued that the findings as to legitimacy were *dicta* and therefore not law.[104] Similar findings were made in *Doornbos v. Doornbos* and in *Gursky v. Gursky* in New York in 1963. A more recent and interesting judgment is *People v. Sorensen* 1968, the only reported decision by an appellate court.[105] This was a criminal prosecution on complaint of the welfare authorities against the husband for failure to support a minor child born, during the marriage, of donor insemination to which he had consented. Without dissent the California Supreme Court held that a child conceived through A.I.D. does not have a "natural" father; the anonymous donor is not the "natural" father; the child does have a lawful father and the defendant was that lawful father. In the court's view:

> In the absence of legislation prohibiting artificial insemination, the offspring of defendant's valid marriage to the child's mother was lawfully begotten. . . .

Finally the court noted:

> Nor are we persuaded that the concept of legitimacy demands that the child be the actual offspring of the husband of the mother and if semen of some other male is utilized the resulting child is illegitimate.

People v. Sorensen has been described as the current leading American case.[106]

"The question of the legitimacy of an A.I.D. child appears never to have been determined by a Canadian or a United Kingdom Court."[107] The absence of court cases may be due to the fact that an A.I.D. child is usually registered in the normal way, at birth, as a legitimate child, although such an action is fraudulent in some jurisdictions. The fact of the A.I.D. origin is not divulged and no one is the wiser about the child's true biological origins. In addition, the common law presumption that the child of a married woman born during the marriage is legitimate unless it is established that the husband was impotent or that it was impossible for the couple to have coitus at the material time operates to prevent any question of the child's legitimacy from arising where husband and wife are cohabiting and continuing to engage in coitus.[108]

Nevertheless, S.E. Kingstone advised the Task Force that "most writers in the absence of any other cases or legislation agree that A.I.D. children are illegitimate."[107]

In the particular case of consensual A.I.D., Lord Kilbrandon, a judge of the House of Lords, the highest court in the United Kingdom, made a valid point when he observed that "the child is legitimate in that it was borne by the wife, in fulfilment of the wishes of the husband, and, in that sense, to call it illegitimate is a misuse of language."[109] There is evidence that some lawyers and judges in Canada concur in his view that the child born of consensual A.I.D. is legitimate.

The Task Force believes that "Christians should work towards getting rid of the conception of illegitimacy as a violation of the personhood of the child so described."[110] If A.I.D. is an acceptable solution for some couples, we think it important that the child's status as a lawful child of the family be accepted, recognized and secured in law.

Birth registration

As for the registration of the child's birth by the parents, unless the presumption that a child born during the marriage is legitimate is rebutted, the child's legal filiation in the common law provinces is as the child of its mother's husband. It would seem then that it should be so registered, a view G.R.B. Whitehead has expressed. [111] The Vital Statistics Acts of Alberta, British Columbia, Manitoba, Nova Scotia, Ontario, P.E.I. and Saskatchewan specifically require a married woman's child to be registered as the husband's child, showing his surname and his particulars. The only exception permitted is if the mother was living separate and apart from her husband at the time of the conception *and* the husband is not the father of the child. If the mother is living with her husband registration of an A.I.D. child would seem to require no departure from the usual. Under the Quebec Civil Code it is also proper to register the child as the husband's legitimate child.

There may be need for legislative amendment of provisions concerning the physician's notice of live birth. Where the notice requires the name of the father and of the mother, a physician knowing A.I.D. had been performed might be reluctant to falsify the entry by naming the husband as the father. The B.C. Royal Commission thus recommended that a new subsection be added to section 3 of the B.C. Vital Statistics Act (RBSC 1962 c.66) requiring the physician in this situation to enter the name of the mother's husband as the name of the father.[112] Where provincial regulations necessitate such change a provision of this nature would clarify the lawfulness of A.I.D. and the child's legal status.

Donor liability

In the consent form, the donor, as the anonymous provider of semen, disclaims all further knowledge of the results, including the identity of the recipient and the fact of the conception of a child. The various consent forms govern the donor-medical practitioner relationship and the practitioner-recipient relationships. They cannot however bind the child born of A.I.D. and hence the donor's signed discharge is not an effective bar to all future inquiry.[113] If the husband subsequently leaves and fails to provide support for the child, and if the child could establish the donor's identity, he might be liable for the child's maintenance, at least in some jurisdictions.[114] Professional confidentiality would seem to bar the likelihood of a child's being able to establish the donor's identity. But the effectiveness of the donor's disclaimer regarding the child has not been tested in the courts.[115] In addition, as already noted, in litigation in Canadian courts, there is no legally protected right to the confidentiality of medical records.

The donor may then, subject to tracing and identification by the child, have the same rights and obligations as the father of an illegitimate child. But the fact that no such cases have yet arisen suggests the probability of pursuit for maintenance is remote.

Support, inheritance and custody

The mother's husband, who consents to A.I.D., should recognize his full responsibility for the support of the child. The consent form which the recipients sign usually includes, and clearly ought to affirm his agreement to recognize the child as his own and heir of his body in all respects including descent of property. Inheritance may pose fewer problems in the future in regard to such children. Recent legislative enactments and judicial decisions tending to make the rights of adopted children equal to those of natural children and to include illegitimate children in the class of children benefiting under wills may suggest a broader, more inclusive concept of family may be beginning to be operative in the succession to property. The B.C. Royal Commission has noted that in view of the donor's anonymity and signed disclaimer regarding the child, neither donor nor child should have any claim of inheritance rights over the other.[116] The question may be raised whether in view of the current broader interpretations of wills some specific protection is needed for the donor.

It is possible but not very likely that difficulties related to custody might arise, for a number of recent judicial decisions in Canada have acceded to the natural father of an illegitimate child rights of access and custody.[117] This trend confirms the need for legal clarification of the status of the mother's husband as the child's father and the recognition of the binding nature of the donor's disclaimer.

Physician liability

In law the physician must exercise a reasonable degree of skill and knowledge in deciding what treatment to give the patient who consults him and in administering this treatment according to professionally approved standards.[118] Although there are no cases involving failure to exercise care in the use of A.I.D., this accepted standard of a reasonable degree of professional care would likely apply to the physician in relation to the selection of appropriate recipients, the administration of insemination and the responsible selection of donors.

There has been concern amongst medico-legal personnel that a higher standard of responsibility might be required of the physician since A.I.D. may be considered a procedure which does not have a curative purpose. (The physician is not curing illness or disability but is fulfilling a patient's desire.) The concern has been expressed that courts might require a physician to be an insurer for any ill results that might be caused by his action even though he could not have prevented these by reasonable care, nor have foreseen the actual consequences.[119]

In recent years, in scattered cases in the U.S., Canada and Australia, courts have awarded compensation to children born alive for damages suffered in utero.[120] Detailed statutes designed to give recompense to children born deformed through injury during pregnancy arising through the acts of a third party are being considered in several countries.[121] If a child created by donor insemination were to be born with defects, the parents or the child itself might well seek tort compensation for negligence from the physician. If he has not exercised reasonable care in selecting a donor and in using known medical procedures and family history questionnaires for genetic investigation of the donor's sperm, or alternatively in selecting a semen bank which employs acceptable screening procedures, he may risk being held negligent. Furthermore, in an appropriate case, the physician might bring third-party proceedings against the donor, for example if he had concealed the fact of a heritable defect.

It is generally believed that the physician and hospitals will be held in Canadian courts to a standard of negligence, rather than to strict liability.[122] The B.C. Royal Commission noted the possibility that implied contractual warranties of product fitness and merchantability derived from the *Sale of Goods Act* might be applied by the courts to the use of semen from a semen bank. With this in mind the commission recommended that the physician fully disclose to the recipient the risks inherent in A.I.D., making sure that she accepts that reasonable care is all that is required of the physician in selecting the donor or semen bank and in performing the insemination, and that the consent form expressly reject any implied warranties.

It should be noted that the consent form may effectively bar an action by the parents but is not an answer to an action by the child who is not party to the agreement. In the light of the problems of liability, the B.C. Royal Commission advised that a new statute should be enacted to impose a negligence standard on the doctor and to expressly exclude any concept of implied warranties.[123]

Doctors at present run the risk of difficulties having to be resolved by the courts. If society is prepared to permit and indeed to subsidize A.I.D. through hospital insurance, it seems reasonable to us that appropriate legislative protection should be accorded to those undertaking to do it.

OTHER SOCIAL POLICY ISSUES

The single woman

The Task Force was asked to consider what response a physician ought to make to requests by single women for A.I.D. Should these by granted? Why, or why not? On what grounds?

Lest it be thought this is borrowing future trouble, Masters and Johnson, recognized American authorities in the field of sexuality, have noted that "unwed motherhood, a status previously accepted out of unhappy necessity, is the deliberate choice of a small but not inconsequential number of women,"[124] and renowned American sociologist Jessie Bernard, who has written widely about both women and marriage, concurs that some respectable women choose motherhood but not marriage.[125]

For its part, the B.C. Royal Commission held that "in principle rules as to eligibility for AID should be the same as for adoption. Thus, it should be possible for a single parent to qualify for this procedure." As reason supporting their stance they asserted that "certainly there are a number of single parent families that are as successful as some in which both parents are present." They recommended that a test of "ability to nurture" focussing on a woman's social and emotional qualities as a prospective parent be developed for use as a guideline by physicians.[126]

We may question first whether the deliberate initiation of pregnancy in a single woman is not in truth a different and greater responsibility than that of giving a child already born into her care. Is adoption really a comparable model?

It would seem that the underlying rationale behind the stance of the B.C. Royal Commission is that fulfilment of feminine nature in childbearing is a basic human right. In Christian understanding of marriage and family, as set forth in the wedding service, bearing a child is a blessing for a married couple and the bearing and care of children belong within the protection of a marital union.[127]

While undeniably there are strong single parent families which might give emotional security to a child, we would observe that the social context does not support such families as well as it does monogamous family units. Certainly society does not offer real support to Lesbian couples.[128]

Pragmatically, we may question with American lawyer Frank P. Grad, "are we ready for the legal problems of assimilating fatherless families . . . into the social fabric?"[129] Such a child would lack the male support which our society seeks to ensure if at all possible and would suffer the legal and social incapacities attendant upon illegitimacy, including social stigma. There is also "a good deal of evidence that [the father's] role in the family is as vital psychologically as that of the mother, and even more so in some stages of the developing ego," in the opinion of Canadian psychiatrists Wendell Watters and J. Sousa-Poza.[130] So such a child might well join the ranks of those whose needs for fathering as they struggle towards maturity are of serious concern to every community and priest. One need only think of the pleas for Big Brothers in every city to shrink from such a policy.

We believe that compassion and prudence alike confirm our understanding that a family with both a mother and a father committed to the child's care is the ideal for which we should strive. We must consider social justice for the child and realize that a child is not only the personal responsibility and fulfilment of its mother but also a concern of the wider community.

Would according A.I.D. to single women imply accepting that a commodity bought through a commercial transaction creates new human life? Until now we have always known a man shared in a child's creation and we may naturally shrink from facing and accepting the new reality. Do our instinctive reactions express an awareness that man-woman partnership is the human way for creating children and ensuring their care, that marriage is the human form of parenthood in the created order? Or is A.I.D. rather a real means of expressing human caring which is not narrowly bound by physical determinism? And is the social solidarity displayed in giving it to a single woman caring enough for the child who is to be born?

Finally, although we are probably talking about a small number of women, is it possible that in this way, through A.I.D., "a dissolvent would be introduced into the social system and the common good seriously damaged"?[131]

Our understanding of family and marriage, and our practical experience thus lead us to reject A.I.D. as a moral option for the single woman. We would urge physicians to reflect seriously on the personal, moral and social values involved in such a practice.

Human semen cryobanking

We have already noted that most of the Task Force think the physician should retain personal responsibility for selecting donors and obtaining semen, since a context of personal accountability seems to offer more control and security. The advent of frozen semen (which has been described as "the refinement that has virtually revolutionized A.I.D."[132]) and of semen banks makes possible a more impersonal and much wider use of donated semen. These also open the door to genetic engineering. Biologists themselves debate the promises in deliberate germinal selection. Some see it as a means for improving the human stock; others hold it would diminish genetic diversity, deny the evolutionary process that has carried us this far and require "a wisdom in the selection of desirable genetic traits which man simply does not possess."[133] Others deny that genetic choice can ensure specific qualities significant to human character, emphasizing instead the complexities and the role of environment. In any case eugenics poses far-reaching moral and practical problems concerning power and who will exercise it, scientific elitism, state control, and, on a deeper level, our understanding of man's creatureliness and freedom and the myths and images by which we will choose to shape humanity's future. All these the church will need to consider when semen cryobanking becomes common.[134]

One physician on the Task Force supports the establishment of a university-based service for frozen semen. Increased resort to A.I.D. in the U.S. has led to a considerable number of commercial semen banks being set up in the last half dozen years, the first being established in 1953 at the University of Iowa. Dr. Kerr noted in 1974 that it was becoming difficult to find enough donors to accommodate the growing numbers of A.I.D. patients seeking his help. If we permit the practice of A.I.D. there seems no prospect of avoiding semen banks and in fact it seems likely that such services must come in Canada in the near future. Indeed Joan Hollobon in the Toronto *Globe and Mail* of June 3, 1976 stated that Dr. Jack Shuber of the Reproductive Biology Unit of Mount Sinai Hospital, Toronto, was looking into the possibilities of setting up such a service.[135] A bank would make a wider variety of semen readily available. At present there is nothing to stop a private commercial semen bank from being established in Canada.[136] The risks in free enterprise in this field seem obvious. We clearly need to ensure the use of adequate standards of donor selection and semen testing, and the best techniques of freezing and storing. In this connection, Charles Feilding noted that the scientific literature submitted to the Task Force indicated there are still serious unanswered technical questions, for instance about the ameliorative or degenerative effects of supercooling on genetic material and the effects of long term storage.[137] There is need to ensure also the use of protective donor consent forms, responsible accessibility for prospective recipients and their physicians, adequate record keeping and confidentiality.[138] In short, consumer protection dictates restriction of semen cryobanking to a unit with the most responsible control, and regulation by some overall authority.

In the light of these needs the B.C. Royal Commission recommended that a service be established on an institutional base and that the Health Protection Branch, Health and Welfare, Canada, should take on responsibility for surveillance of human semen banking, with associated collection, processing, distribution and documentation services, under a mandate which would require federal legislation.[139] Although most of the Task Force does not favour semen banks, in the event they are to be established we consider the B.C. recommendations suggest a prudent policy.

EMBRYO TRANSFER

The Task Force had originally intended to deal with the complex ethical, social and legal aspects of embryo transfer. But we have concluded that to treat these adequately will require another study.[140]

In vitro fertilization — the fertilization outside a woman's body of an ovum — and the growth of a human embryo to blastocyst stage had been reported by 1971. July 15, 1974 newspapers around the world excitedly flashed a report from English doctor D.C.A. Bevis that a number of children, some as old as 18 months, had already been born following transfer of an embryo back into its mother's body. No subsequent confirmation has been published in scientific journals and as of March 15, 1975, the *Medical Journal of Australia* stated: "It must be stressed that the age of embryo transfer is not yet upon us since, at the time of going to press, no report of a successful embryo transfer between human beings has yet appeared."[141] In the winter of 1975-76, apparently neither English scientist R.G. Edwards nor American physician Landrum Shettles, leading figures involved in this research, had any success to report and both appeared to be at a standstill in their work.[142]

Scientists and physicians emphasize that embryo transfer is being sought to enable a woman and her husband to bear their own child, in cases where blocked tubes prevent the woman from conceiving through normal sexual intercourse. It appears to be proving more difficult than anticipated to obtain the endocrine conditions required to sustain the life of the transferred embryo while employing prior treatment to secure oocytes, by laparoscopy, at the right stage of maturation. It seems clear that ultimately the work will be successful. Provided one accepts that use of techniques does not seriously threaten human personality and risk dehumanization, there is less moral difficulty about the transfer to a woman of her own and her husband's germinal material; they contribute more equally to the creation of their future child than in the A.I.D. situation. But Dr. Kerr has pointed out that only a minority of women with blocked tubes can provide their own eggs, since many have ovarian adhesions. Thus donor eggs will be required. He has also urged "we must accept the corollary that development will not stop at the management of the subfertile woman."[143] The moral issues related to the use of donor eggs, foster wombs for the fetus' growth, genetic engineering to breed for quality, and perhaps later asexual reproduction by cloning will certainly arise out of successful embryo transfer and will have to be confronted. We will have to face up to the challenge of balancing the risks which biomedical technology poses of depersonalization and of vastly increased power of scientists over the fabric of human life, against the possibilities of authentic human fulfilment on wider and deeper levels. We will then indeed have to think deeply about human values and apply them with great care and responsibility to a wide range of issues related to embryo transfer.

TASK FORCE CONCLUSIONS

Ethical issues

1. The Task Force is divided on whether A.I.D. is fully acceptable morally and whether it is socially desirable.

2. None of us considers that A.I.D. is clearly morally wrong, nor do we believe it should be made illegal or unavailable. We know of no certain evidence that A.I.D. causes personal hurt to couples, nor since it is practised on a small scale, does it pose a threat to the common good.

3. We believe that A.I.D. given to a wife by a qualified physician, with the consent of her husband, should not be considered in either morals or law to be adultery.

4. The child born following such A.I.D. should be considered the child of the husband and wife and should have full legal standing as a lawful child of their family.

5. The majority of us believe that A.I.D. for a woman whose husband is sterile or genetically unfit to give her a healthy child may be a fully acceptable medical treatment. It seems to us to be a humane response to a legitimate human need which in the absence of readily adoptable children cannot at present be met in any other way. We accept it largely because we see children as a precious and real fulfillment of a couple's love, and in faithfulness to the belief which Christians share with many others that children are a blessing enriching marriage and society.

6. Some of us have serious personal reservations about A.I.D., based on our understanding of Christian teachings about marriage and about human nature. Holding that for Christians marriage is a joining, before God, of two persons in a mutual life, we believe that a married couple denied the blessing of children may yet live creatively in true self-giving, and together find fulfilment as they serve God by reflecting his love within the family of man. And we believe that, given the psychosomatic unity of persons, the creation of new life should be by a husband and wife in the personal intimacy of sexual union.*

7. Some of us believe there is an important human value in the acceptance by a man of full responsibility for the life which his sperm creates. We personally have doubts about the morality of semen donation.*

8. The others believe that, where A.I.D. is responsibly undertaken, men may legitimately be confident that the child which their sperm may create is wanted and will be cared for, and that their donation of sperm is humane and responsible.

9. Some of us believe that in the light of the reality that women are only now being encouraged to discover an independent identity, neither church nor society ought to stress that woman's fulfilment lies only or chiefly in maternity. Since we are also confronted with the urgent need to deal with world-wide problems of poverty and social injustice, resource depletion, overpopulation and pollution, we wonder if the church has a responsibility to refrain from building social pressures on couples to have children.

10. We believe that A.I.D. should not be given to single women. We think that while many single women are successfully raising children alone, having a father is nevertheless very important to a child. It is unwise and unjust deliberately to create a child who can have no expectation of having a father. Those of us who are priests know that women and their fatherless

*Phyllis Creighton, Eugene Fairweather, Charles Feilding, Paul Gibson, David McCallion.

children frequently show great need of male support which it is difficult to find in our society.

Medical aspects

11. A.I.D. may pose a threat to a man's self-image, since it involves acceptance of his inability to create a child and the fulfilment of his and his wife's needs and their desire for her to bear a child in spite of this. Therefore, in our opinion, a physician should ensure that those seeking A.I.D. have careful counselling and should select for the procedure only mature couples who have fully come to terms with their feelings and whose marriage shows the strengths needed to cope with the extra psychological burden which A.I.D. imposes.

12. A professional team including both male and female members, for instance a physician and a nurse practitioner, and possibly other experts such as a psychiatrist or social worker experienced in marital or adoption problems, may be of real value for this kind of service.

13. We think it is important that donors be carefully selected, with a view to eliminating those with serious medical or genetic risk, or undesirable motivation. They should be personally convinced that semen donation is a responsible act.

14. Since there is much more A.I.D. now than just a few years ago, more extended follow-up studies of the families involved could usefully be undertaken, in our opinion, in order to confirm selection criteria, to learn more about the development of personal relationships in such families, and to discover problems that might be avoided or ways of dealing with them.

15. The Task Force reached no consensus on the meaning and risks of the secrecy with which most of those involved in A.I.D. believe it should be surrounded and the value of full honesty and openness in the A.I.D. situation. Some of us think the present stance makes sense in today's circumstances, to protect persons from hurt. Others question whether the insistence on secrecy indicates that conflicts about the process have not been entirely worked through, and consider that greater honesty and openness would create a more supportive atmosphere for A.I.D. couples and their families.

16. It seems likely to us that some A.I.D. children will discover the nature of their conception and may experience an identity crisis in which certainty about their biological origins is important. We therefore believe that full medical records of the donors, using a suitable coding system to protect individuals, should be kept, so that a child may later be helped, through informed counselling, to come to terms with himself or herself.

Legal concerns

17. Our basic stance concerning the law is predicated on the views expressed in points 3 and 4, that consensual A.I.D. should not be considered adultery and that the child born following such A.I.D. should be considered the child of the consenting couple.

18. We have discovered that there is uncertainty about the legal implications of A.I.D. because of conflicting judgments in legal cases and the absence of specific statutory rulings. Clearly there are important interests of the recipient couples, their families, the donor, and the medical practitioner, to be protected. To minimize risks to these persons, and to prevent the possibility of adverse decisions, it would seem that legal doubts about the effect of A.I.D. on the status of both the marriage and the child should be removed by legislative enactment. This might be done by amendment to existing legislation. In the provinces, the various statutes dealing with the status of children might provide that children born as the result of A.I.D. undertaken with the consent of the husband have the same status as children born within the marriage in the normal way. The *Divorce Act*, 1968, a federal statute, could be amended to provide that A.I.D. with the consent of the husband, not constitute adultery. Preferably, as in some other jurisdictions, the whole subject of A.I.D. should be a matter for legislative enactment.

19. We agree that if society is prepared to permit A.I.D., it should accord appropriate legislative protection to those undertaking to do it. In the light of the existing uncertainty concerning the physician's liability in A.I.D. and of the risks inherent in leaving the issues to be resolved by the courts, we think that there should be legislation to impose a negligence standard on the physician in the matter of A.I.D.

20. Most of the Task Force think it preferable that the individual physician retain control of semen donation, in order to ensure careful selection of donors. In the light of the growing demand for A.I.D. it seems likely, however, that frozen human semen banks will be established. We think that government regulations need to be devised to ensure that such facilities have reasonable and medically acceptable standards for selection of donors, preservation and storage of semen, access to its use, securing of consent, and record keeping. The risks in unregulated commercial enterprise in this field make protection for the public necessary.

APPENDIX

Reprinted from the *Ninth Report of the Royal Commission on Family and Children's Law; Artificial Insemination* (Vancouver, May 1975), Appendix III A, B.

AGREEMENT — DONOR

WHEREAS:

I, ______________________________, have been given the opportunity to donate my semen for the purpose of artificial insemination of a woman whose identity is unknown to me, and would wish to have protection of my interests and those of all concerned;

THEREFORE:

1. I acknowledge that I understand the purpose of such artificial insemination is to produce a child or children.

2. I acknowledge that I do not expect to have divulged to me the identity of the said woman, her husband, or of the child or children who may be produced as the result of such insemination, nor do I expect to learn whether such insemination(s) do indeed result in the birth of a child or children.

3. I agree not to seek out the identity of the said child or children, nor of either of the parents.

4. I understand that no consideration will be given to the religion of either the donor or the recipient.

5. I take full responsibility for any decision to inform any of my own relatives of this semen donation and its purpose, or to withold such information, and full responsibility for any actual or alleged effects that this donation may have on any of them, with the understanding that my identity will not be divulged to the woman or women inseminated by my semen, nor to her marital partner, nor to any child or children conceived by such insemination(s). In fact, I donate my semen with the agreement that the doctor who is responsible for this collection undertakes to keep my identity confidential, and unknown to anyone except those directly involved in the collection.

6. I agree to submit to a standard physical examination and to any tests which are explained to me for the detection of any inheritable disease or other defect, and to supply true and full answers to the said doctor in connection with questions bearing upon heritable or communicable diseases in myself or relatives, or risk thereof. It is my understanding that such information will be treated in confidence, and not linked to my identity in any documents outside the confidential files of the doctor responsible for the semen collection.

7. It has been explained that any financial or other compensation I may receive will be restricted to considerations such as the expenditure of my time, loss of income or travel expense caused by my donation.

WHEREFORE:

The donor and doctor have hereto set their hands and seals this ____________ day of ____, A.D. 19 ____.

Donor ______________

Place ______________ Doctor ______________

AGREEMENT — RECIPIENT FAMILY

WHEREAS:

______________ and ______________,
husband and wife, desire to engage the services of Dr.
______________, ______________,
or ______________, of ______________,

to perform one or more, if necessary, artificial insemination procedures with sperm from a stranger donor, and it is desired that an agreement be made in order to fully protect the interests of the husband, wife, the child who may be the issue of such artificial insemination, the donor, the doctor(s), and any laboratory used in supplying the sperm:

THEREFORE:

1. The husband and the wife hereby acknowledge that they understand that the purpose of the insemination is to attempt to produce a pregnancy in the wife, that any pregnancy involves the risk of a miscarriage or other complications, difficulties in delivery and birth defects, and that the risk of such problems is also present in pregnancies resulting from artificial insemination.

2. It is agreed by and between the above named husband and wife that the said doctor is hereby engaged to perform the procedure of artificial insemination upon the wife, the said doctor to obtain the necessary sperm from a donor who shall not be advised of the identity of the said husband and wife, nor of the success or failure of the insemination, and who shall agree in writing not to seek out the identity of the said husband or wife, nor of any child who may be the issue of such insemination. Furthermore, the said husband and wife acknowledge that the identity of the said donor is not to be divulged to them, and they agree not to seek out his identity.

3. The husband and wife hereby authorize the doctor, in his sole and absolute discretion, to use fresh or frozen semen from one or more such unidentified donor(s), to select the donor(s), and to select the laboratory which has collected, processed and stored frozen semen.

4. It is understood that the religion of neither the donor nor of the recipient or her spouse will be considered in selecting the donor.

5. The husband and wife hereby fully agree that each understands that the doctor cannot be responsible for the physical or mental characteristics of any child so produced; and do hereby absolve and release the doctor, his collaborating colleagues, the institution in which he practices, the donor(s), and the laboratory involved in sperm collection from any liability of whatever kind and nature arising out of, resulting from, or in collection and processsing of semen or from any other aspect of the artificial insemination procedure.

6. It is further agreed that, at the moment of conception, the said husband hereby accepts the conception as though it were the result of his own marital act, and agrees: (a) that such child or children so produced are his own legally produced child or children and are the heirs of his body, and (b) that he hereby completely waives forever any right which he might have to disclaim such child or children as his own, and (c) that such child or children so produced are, and shall be considered to be, in all respects, including descent of property, child or children of his own body.

7. And it is further agreed by the said wife that in all legal aspects, the said husband shall be considered as the father of such child or children.

8. It is further agreed that the nature of this agreement is such that it must remain confidential and, therefore, the husband and wife agree that the sole copy of the same may be given to the said doctor for his confidential files.

WHEREFORE:

The said doctor, husband and wife have hereto set their hands and seals this ___ day of ________, A.D. 19____.

Husband ______________

Place ________________ Wife ______________

NOTES

1. The technique of insemination was first successfully used with a husband's semen in England at the end of the 18th century. Donor insemination is reported to have been used first in the U.S. in 1884. (A.T. Gregoire and R.C. Mayer, "The impregnators," *Fertility and Sterility*, 16 (1965), 130-34). Artificial insemination with husband's semen (A.I.H.) is now infrequently used but is still of some value. The Church of England in 1948 held that suitably chosen couples might legitimately use it. It affirmed that moral concern about the masturbation required for semen collection could be resolved by the judgment that the process as a whole was directed to a legitimate end of marriage. A.I.H. can be of value in certain rare instances of anatomical or functional disturbances of ejaculation. Where impotence is the difficulty it is almost always preferable to deal with the personal and sexual problems of the couple. In his paper for the Task Force Dr. Kerr noted there is continuing interest in its use where a husband's ejaculates have small numbers of spermatozoa; these can be pooled, using freezing methods which preserve their activity, and the larger pooled volume used for A.I.H. Although publicity has recently been given to such attempts, he considers there is still little evidence to support expectations of successful insemination. A published version of his paper may be consulted. *See* M. G. Kerr and Carol Rogers, "Donor insemination," *Journal of Medical Ethics* (London), I (April 1975), 30-33.

2. Alun Jones and W.F. Bodner, *Our future inheritance: choice or chance?* (London, 1974), 16.

3. The Task Force has expressed its concern about the seriousness of recourse to abortion in *Abortion, an issue for conscience* (Toronto, 1974).

4. Betty Graham, in "Some comments respecting adoption and A.I.D.," (a Task Force paper in General Synod Archives, Anglican Church of Canada, Toronto) noted that in Ontario over 5,000 children were placed annually by Children's Aid Societies in the peak years 1968-69-70, (1969: 5,477), but in 1972 there were only 3,260 and in 1975 the figure dropped to 2,187. She indicated a similar pattern was reported in B.C. in 1973.

5. See *Globe and Mail* (Toronto), 5 Dec. 1974, Kathleen Rex, "These children come wrapped in red tape," page W 1.

6. C. R. Feilding, 25 February 1974 paper for the Task Force in the Archives of Anglican Church of Canada, Toronto.

7. "Annual report of Council: Appendices, Appendix V: Report of panel on human artificial insemination," *British Medical Journal (Supplement)*, 2 (April 7, 1973), 3-5, at para. (13).

8. Articles in *Homemaker's Digest* Jan-Feb. 1972; *Good Housekeeping*, Jan. 1973; *Chatelaine*, Sept. 1975; *Globe and Mail*, 2,3,5 June 1976; CTV's W5 program 20 June 1976, all indicate growing interest.

9. It is difficult to know how far medical approval reflects public attitudes. When the Peel panel published its report, (cited in footnote 7 supra), a *Times* editorial expressing severe reserve concluded: "Next time there is a committee appointed to reconsider human artificial insemination it had better include a layman or two." See Horace Krever, "Some legal implications of advances in human genetics," *Canadian Journal of Genetics and Cytology*, XVII (3)(Sept. 1975), 283-96, at 285. Alun Jones and W.F. Bodmer, *op. cit.* in footnote 2 supra, 23, state that the subject is discussed more freely and with less repugnance, but in 1974 there was "still no apparent widespread call in Britain for A.I.D. to be provided under the National Health Service."

10. *Good Housekeeping*, January 1973, 73, 127-29, carried a deeply moving personal account of a husband's struggle to come to terms with his infertility, fears and longings, and to choose A.I.D. The turning point in his numbing despair came when he realized that "I was a man whose gift of life need not be dependent on any power to produce genetic particles encoded to create a copy of myself. I would be able to find myself continued in the chain of life not by a certain color of eyes or hair, but by the day-to-day process of giving to a child all that I could — my knowledge, my support, my joy in discovery, my love." The man "frustrated in his faith in blood-and-genes procreation began changing into a man whose feeling of self-worth lay in the confidence that he could be as much or more of a father to his children as any other man." (At page 128).

11. *op. cit.*, 14-17.

12. *ibid*, 58.

13. *ibid*, 51.

14. *ibid*, 58.

15. *ibid*, 31.

16. *ibid*, 61.

17. *ibid*, 60-62.

18. See Norman St. John-Stevas, *Life, death and the law: a study of the relationship between law and Christian morals in the English and American legal systems* (London 1961), 142. He notes, 138,139, that the Roman Catholic Church, in speeches made by Pius XII Sept. 29, 1949, October 29, 1951 and May 19, 1956, also rejected A.I.D.

19. *Report of the departmental committee on human artificial insemination* (Home Office, Scottish Home Department, London, 1960), rec. 123.

20. recs. 264, 268.

21. *ibid*, 83, 85.

22. *Ninth report of the Royal Commission on Family and Children's Law: artificial insemination* (Vancouver, 1975), 8.

23. Paul Gibson, "Is artificial insemination by donor adultery?", paper written for the Task Force, in the Archives of the Anglican Church of Canada, Toronto.

24. Genesis 2: 21-25; Mark 10: 2-12; Ephesians 5: 25-33.

25. Charles Feilding also suggested, in his paper of 25 Feb. 1974, that we are at a turning point in current theological discussion where mutual love and comfort will be seen as the primary end of an individual marriage and procreation will be understood as an important optional end. Canon XXI puts mutual fellowship first and "the procreation (if it may be) and nurture of children" second as purposes of marriage.

26. C. E. Curran, *Politics, medicine and Christian ethics: a dialogue with Paul Ramsey* (Philadelphia, 1973), 217.

27. According to Task Force member Richard Roach, S.J., it was held that "nature or natural law has joined that physical causality [of the generation of new life] to the interpersonal relationship of a man and a woman which we call marriage in such a way that it is immoral to separate them." See his paper "Nature: norm or challenge," (typescript for the Task Force, in the Archives of the Anglican Church of Canada, Toronto), in which the material in this paragraph and the previous one was critically developed.

28. Genesis 16: 1-4.

29. Joseph Fletcher, *Morals and Medicine* ... (Princeton, N.J., 1954), 139.

30. Massimo Piattelli-Palmarini, "Biological roots of the human individual", *Law and ethics of A.I.D. and embryo transfer*, Ciba Foundation Symposium 17 (new series) (Amsterdam and New York, 1973) 19-25, at page 21. This book will be cited as CIBA *Symposium* 17 (1973) in footnotes hereafter.

31. Anglican moral theologian G.R. Dunstan sees the view of A.I.D. as a technical intervention as a "cerebral judgement" and suggests that whether it "does justice to the whole socio-psycho-physical reality of the problem ... requires close discussion in the light of ... research." CIBA *Symposium* 17 (1973), 51-52.

32. Dunstan thinks it withdraws biological from personal potential and reverses "the long process of evolution by which biological capacities have been humanized." He implies that by his understanding of human nature and values it might be a less than human act to which love, as the final purpose, could not therefore oblige a man. *ibid.* Dr. Kerr has advised that G.R. Dunstan has published more recent comments in a report of a workshop held in Nov. 1976 on artificial insemination which has just been issued (1977) by the Royal College of Obstetricians and Gynaecologists, London.

33. Eugene Fairweather, "Natural law as ethical norm: some principles and problems," paper for the Task Force, in the Archives of the Anglican Church of Canada, Toronto.

34. Rosemary Haughton in "Theology of marriage," in *Male and Female: Christian approaches to sexuality* (New York, 1976), a recent publication of the Episcopal Church, stresses, at page 221, the Christian view that the "actions of the body pull the spiritual, essential person". This view contrasts with the notion, widely held in our society, that man is directed by reason and will, the mind being conceived as the driver of the "car," the body.

35. Joseph Fletcher, *op. cit.* at footnote 29 supra, 127.

36. Karl Ostrom, "Psychological considerations in evaluating A.I.D." in "An interdisciplinary case study — Artificial insemination donor: a simple medical technique, a complex human problem," *Soundings, an interdisciplinary journal,* LIV (1971), 288-343, at page 296.

37. Helmut Thielicke, *The Ethics of Sex* (New York, Evanston and London, 1964), 257.

38. Joseph Fletcher, *op. cit.* at footnote 29 supra, 117.

39. *See* Van Rensselaer Potter, "The ethics of nature and nurture," *New Theology No. 10,* edited by M.E. Marty and D.G. Peerman (New York and London, 1973), 38-53.

40. Josef Fuchs, *Human values and Christian morality* (Dublin and London, 1970), 115-17, 143, 183-84. See also G.R. Dunstan, *The artifice of ethics, the Moorhouse lectures 1973* (London, 1974), especially chapter 4, "Born to rule", 56-73, for a discussion of various theologians' views of nature and the ethics of medical intervention in reproduction.

41. Eugene Fairweather, paper cited in footnote 33 supra.

42. C.E. Curran, *Contemporary problems in moral theology*, (Notre Dame, Ind., 1970), 215.

43. L.R. Kass expresses fears about the dehumanization through new reproductive techniques in "New beginnings in life", in *The new genetics and the future of man*, edited by M.P. Hamilton (Grand Rapids, Michigan, 1972), 15-63.

44. R.G. Edwards, "Fertilization of human eggs in vitro: morals, ethics and the law," *Quarterly Review of Biology* 49 (March 1974), 3-26, at page 15.

45. Personal comment of T.B. Robson, M.D., obstetrician, member of the Task Force.

46. *Changing man: the threat and the promise; five scientists and five theologians on Christian faith and evolutionary thought,* edited by Kyle Haselden and Philip Hefner (Garden City, N.Y., 1968), 26.

47. *3 issues in ethics*, (New York, 1970), 79.

48. At one major Ontario university hospital donors receive $25 per sperm sample.

49. See R. Schoysman, "Problems of selecting donors for artificial insemination," *Journal of Medical Ethics* (London) I (April 1975), 34-38.

50. CIBA *Symposium* 17 (1973), 31.

51. Program of Policy Studies in Science and Technology, George Washington University, Monograph No. 18, December 1973, at pp. 22-23.

52. *op. cit.*, rec. 11 at p. 16-17.

53. *ibid.*, rec. 9 at p. 15.

54. D.A. Goss, "Current status of artificial insemination with donor semen", *American Journal of Obstetrics and Gynecology* 122 (2) (15 May 1975): 246-52, at 250, notes pre-ovulatory mucus must exhibit adequate ferning and spinnbarkheit, which can be assessed.

55. D.A. Goss, *ibid*, at 250, recently reported 63% success rate with normal patients, 46% with those requiring treatment for some pathological condition.

56. Our medical data and Dr. Kerr's statements, where not footnoted, are published in the article he co-authored which is cited in footnote 1 supra. See also his March 1977 paper for the Royal College of Physicians and Surgeons (London), "Counselling and selection of recipients for A.I.D.," in the Archives of the Anglican Church of Canada, Toronto.

57. M.G. Kerr, *op. cit.* in footnote 1 Supra.

58. J.H. Edwards, British geneticist, suggested at the 1972 CIBA Symposium, that it is difficult to establish infertility with certainty. See CIBA *Symposium* 17 (1973), p. 28. On the other hand, A.T. Himmelweit expressed concern that as A.I.D. is a simple technique, it might be too quickly given without thorough investigation of the male's infertility problem; *ibid.*, 102. Dr. Kerr thinks that in the current primitive state of our ability to assess male fertility, substantial emphasis should be put on the couple's reproductive history.

59. Dr. Kerr gave the examples of cancer, especially testicular cancer, treatment for cancer or some kidney diseases, severe diabetes, paraplegia.

60. D.A. Goss, *op. cit.*, in footnote 54 supra, at p. 247, however holds that the man's ill health or doubt about the longevity of his life rule out A.I.D.

61. M.G. Kerr, *op. cit.* in footnote 1 supra.

62. Barbara Ehrenreich and Deirdre English, *Complaints and disorders: the sexual politics of sickness,* Glass Mountain pamphlet No. 2, the Feminist Press (New York, 1973), 83. *See* also Diana Scully and Pauline Barr, "A funny thing happened on the way to the orifice: women in gynecology textbooks," *American Journal of Sociology* 78 (4) (January 1973), 1045-50.

63. Interestingly, D.A. Goss, *op. cit.*, at footnote 54 supra, at page 249, points out that many referring physicians have expressed their reluctance to be placed in this role which they see as unique and entailing heavy responsibilities.

64. Joan Holland, "Adoption and artificial insemination: some social implications," in article and issue of *Soundings* cited at footnote 36 supra, 302-27, at 303.

65. Frankel, *op. cit.*, at footnote 51 supra, 14.

66. *See* Titmuss's book, *The gift relationship: from human blood to social policy* (London, 1970), 151.

67. The semen donor interviewed on CTV's W5, 20 June 1976, displayed a supercilious pride in the fact that he and those he recruited for semen donation were of superior intelligence; his attitude validated the kinds of skeptical questions raised in the 1948 Church of England report, *Artificial human insemination,* at 27-28. G. R. Dunstan, CIBA *Symposium* 17 (1973), 52, agrees there is "a regrettable ignorance and uncertainty about his motives . . . about the effects of his action upon himself . . . and about his suitability . . . for the role of progenitor of a child to which he will remain for ever unrelated."

68. at page 23.

69. Bridgett Mason, Royal Free Hospital, London, infertility clinic, quoted in CIBA *Symposium* 17 (1973), 57-58.

70. rec. 12. M.S. Frankel in *op. cit.* in footnote 51 supra, at page 46, noted in the literature a reference to one donor siring 35 offspring.

71. appendix III A, reprinted in the appendix of this volume.

72. rec. 7.

73. Church of England report, *Artificial human insemination*, 53.

74. P.J. Graham in CIBA *Symposium* 17 (1973), 65.

75. Joan Holland, *op. cit.*, at footnote 64 supra, 305.

76. as Holland sees it, *ibid.*, 304.

77. *Utopian motherhood, new trends in human reproduction:* (Garden City, N.Y. 1970), 20.

78. Anne McLaren, CIBA *Symposium* 17 (1973), 67.

79. Legal clarification of the donor's responsibility where A.I.D. is performed on a woman without her husband's consent would also seem to be essential, unless this use of insemination is statutorily declared unlawful.

80. "Family engineers recommend keeping the father a secret," *Globe and Mail*, 3 June 1976.

81. H.W. Horne, Jr., "Artificial insemination, donor: an issue of ethical and moral values," *New England Journal of Medicine* 293 (17) (23 Oct. 1975), 873-74.

82. at page 52.

83. Jo Carson, " 'Even if she's a drunk, I want to meet mother'," *Globe and Mail*, 18 March 1976.

84. "No secrets: adopted get help in Britain," *Globe and Mail,* 21 Oct. 1976. On the Canadian situation regarding adoption and information, see June Callwood, "Adoption not all hearts and flowers," *Chatelaine*, April 1976, 106-13.

85. The right to information is a particularly thorny problem in A.I.D. since it might have serious implications for the donor. British scientist R.G. Edwards noted difficulties have arisen in Germany. "A.I.D. has become acceptable ethically and legally in Germany . . . but recently unexpected legal complexities were revealed since the child is not a party to any agreement between the infertile couple, the doctor, and semen donor; the child could claim damages from the doctor for withholding the identity of its natural father . . . . If the doctor is to be safeguarded as fully as possible, the identity of the semen donor must be clear beyond doubt, his wife must consent, the infertile couple should be aware of the legal difficulties, and the donor must be aware that the offspring can demand to know his name and claim him as its natural father. Many doctors and donors will obviously be dissuaded from A.I.D. by these demands." Edwards also suggested "a parallel situation is arising in the United Kingdom, where adoption agencies and sponsors of a current Parliamentary Bill are pressing for changes in the law to give adopted children the right of access to their original birth certificate. . . . " *op. cit.* in footnote 44 supra, at page 17-18.

86. *Globe and Mail, op. cit.* in footnote 80 supra, 3 June 1976.

87. J.O. Haman, 216 couples, *California Medicine* 90 (1959), 130-33; L.H. Levie, 58 couples, *Eugenics Review* LIX (1967), 97-105; G. Langer, E. Lemberg, and M. Sharf, 156 couples, *International Journal of Fertility* 14 (July-Sept. 1969), 232-40; R.C. Strickler, D.W. Keller, J.C. Warren, 141 patients, *New England Journal of Medicine* 293 (17) (1975), 848-53. See also W.W. Watters and J. Sousa-Poza, "Psychiatric aspects of artificial insemination (donor)," *Canadian Medical Association Journal* 95 (16 July 1966), 106-13.

88. *Globe and Mail, op. cit.* in footnote 80 supra, 3 June 1976.

89. rec. 33. It noted it had been urged by several sources that for psychological reasons there should be no follow-up of children born of A.I.D. It also suggested in rec. 31 that the donor's anonymity could be preserved by keeping information in coded form.

90. Oklahoma, Georgia and California have statutes legalizing A.I.D., and New York city has public health regulations related to it. Similar legislation has been rejected in the U.K., Virginia, Wisconsin, Indiana, Minnesota and New York state, according to Lillian Atallah, "New York becoming 'test-tube' capital," *Globe and Mail*, 5 June 1976.

91. *Ontario Law Reports* 49 (1921), 15-27, at page 22-23.

92. "Artificial insemination", *Canadian Bar Review* 34, 11-27, at page 16.

93. *Scots Law Times: Reports* (1958), 12-18, at page 17.

94. Olive Stone, "English law in relation to A.I.D. and embryo transfer," CIBA *Symposium* 17 (1973), 69, footnote 2. She mentions that *Dennis v. Dennis* [1955] 2 All E.R. (*The All England Law Reports*), 51 C.A., also held that sexual intercourse involved penetration.

95. *Russell v. Russell* [1924] *Appeal Cases*, 687, House of Lords, the case which gave rise to the well-known judgment, at 721, that "fecundation ab extra is, I doubt not, adultery"; *Sapsford v. Sapsford and Furtado,* [1954] 2 All E.R. 373.

96. K. R.M. Hennessy, "Artificial insemination," *Canadian Bar Journal* 10 (1967), 514-23 at 519.

97. Olive Stone, *op. cit.*, at footnote 94 supra, 69.

98. S.E. Kingstone, "A.I.D. — some legal factors," paper for the Task Force, Oct. 1973, in Archives of the Anglican Church of Canada, Toronto.

99. *Scots Law Times: Reports* (1958), at page 14. In a subsequent debate on the matter in the House of Lords, Lord Denning, the Master of the Rolls, the judge who presides over the English Court of Appeal, went further. He contended that if A.I.D. was done without the husband's knowledge or consent, it was "a fraud and an unlawful, indictable conspiracy." He condemned it as a double unlawful conspiracy, first of the doctor with the wife (to keep secret the fact that a child is illegitimate and falsely pretend it is legitimate), and secondly, of the doctor with the donor (to keep his act secret so he might evade the responsibilities to maintain his own child which by law attach to him). See *Law and Morality*, edited by Louis Blom-Cooper and Gavin Drewry (London, 1976), 174-75.

100. "Legal approaches to the new biology," *Population and the new biology*, edited by Bernard Benjamin *et al* (London and New York, 1974), 159-76, at 166.

101. Another problem is the possibility that the birth of an A.I.D. child may not constitute a consummation of the marriage. For this reason the B. C. Royal Commission recommended that A.I.D. should not be a basis for an allegation that there has been a failure to consummate the marriage. Rec. 1.

102. 78 N.Y. Supplement, 2d Ser., 390.

103. *ibid.*, at 391-92.

104. In "Artificial insemination," *Canadian Bar Review* 34 (1956), 166-86, at 169.

105. 68 Cal.2d 280, 66 Cal. Rptr. 7, 437 P.2d 495, 25 *American Law Reports* 3d 1093.

106. *In the matter of the adoption of anonymous, a minor under the age of fourteen (14) years,* 345 N. Y. Supplement 2d. Ser., 430. See 433.

107. S.E. Kingstone, *op cit.* in footnote 98 supra.

108. G.R.B. Whitehead, a lawyer who was then practising in Quebec, asserted that under the Quebec Civil Code, art. 218, the A.I.D. child is the husband's legitimate child, although if the insemination was done without his consent, or if he was either impotent or in the physical impossibility of meeting his wife at the time the child was conceived, he might, within certain restrictive time limits, disown it under articles 219 and 220. See his article, "Artificial insemination and the law," *Chitty's Law Journal* 15 (1967), 218-23, at 221.

109. CIBA *Symposium* 17 (1973), 92.

110. Charles Feilding, 25 Feb. 1974 paper for the Task Force.

111. *op. cit.*, in footnote 108 supra, at 221.

112. rec. 17.

113. D.J. Cusine, "A.I.D. and the law," *Journal of Medical Ethics*, I (April 1975), 39-41, at page 41.

114. The B. C. Royal Commission notes the *Children of Unmarried Parents Act* would apply there, at page 5.

115. B.M. Dickens, *op. cit.*, at footnote 100 supra, 167.

116. rec. 13.

117. S.E. Kingstone advises: access may be given to the putative father, see: *Re Crespy* (1970), 3 *Reports on Family Law* 124 (Ont. C.A.); *Re Leeson* (1971), 5 R.F.L. 46 (B.C. S.C.); *Sobel v. Fogler* (1972), 6 R.F.L. 198 (Ont. S.C.); *White v. Barrett* (1973), 10 R.F.L. 90 (Alta. S.C.). Custody may be given to the putative father, see: *Re Sheppard* (1972), 5 R.F.L. 371 (N.S. C.Ct.); *Re Staples* (1971) 6 R.F.L. 278 (B.C. S.C.); *Misfeldt v. Chowen (Shapansky) and Chowen* (1973), 9 R.F.L. 360 (Sask. Q.B.); *Re West* (1972) 9 R.F.L. 382 (N.S. S.C.); *Re Adams* (1975). 22 R.F.L. 321 (Sask. Q.B.)

118. Halsbury.

119 Letter from the Canadian Medical Protective Association, 22 Jan. 1974.

120. *Duval et al v. Seguin et al, Ontario Reports* 2 (1972), 686. See also A.J. Quinn and J.A. Griffin, "The rights of the unborn," *The Jurist* 31 (1971), 577-613, especially 590-600.

121 R.G. Edwards, *op. cit.*, in footnote 44 supra, 16.

122. A. M. Linden, "The negligent doctor," *Osgoode Hall Law Journal 11* (1973), 31-39.

123. rec. 15.

124 W.H. Masters and V.E. Johnson, *The pleasure bond: a new look at sexuality and commitment* (Boston, 1975), 179.

125 *Women, wives, mothers: values and options* (Chicago, 1975), 70. It is interesting to note that radical feminists Phyllis Chesler and Shulamith Firestone believe science should be used to release woman entirely from the oppression of biological reproduction. See Chesler's *Women and Madness* (New York, 1972), 294, and S. Firestone's *The dialectic of sex: the case for feminist revolution* (New York 1971), 44-45.

126 pp. 10-11, and rec. 3.

127 St. John-Stevas contends that for Christians "the argument that every woman has a "right" to bear a child has no validity, for outside of the married state no such claim is recognized." See *op. cit.*, in footnote 18 supra, 137.

128 Lesbian mothers can face a heavy burden through society's disapproval of homosexuality. Bettie Wysor in *The Lesbian Myth* (New York, 1974), 345, quotes a Lesbian mother that "to carry both the children and this life style — and the life that we have to go through — it's just a heavy thing, and so we just tend to resent it."

129. F.P. Grad, "Legislative responses to the new biology: limits and possibilities," *UCLA Law Rev.* 15 (1968), 480-509, at page 493.

130. *op. cit.*, at footnote 87 supra, 111. They go on to say the father's physical absence from the family has long been associated with serious forms of social pathology, such as delinquency.

131 St. John-Stevas, *op. cit.*, in footnote 18 supra, 144.

132. Lillian Atallah, "No longer a mystery, artificial insemination still causes ethical, legal problems," *Globe and Mail*, 2 June 1976.

133. C.P. Kindregan, "State power over human fertility and individual liberty," *Hastings Law Journal* 23 (1971-72), 1401-26 at 1413, citing P. Medawar, R. Dubos, T. Dobzhansky and others.

134. See James Reed, "Knowledge, power, man and justice: ethical problems in biomedical research," *Canadian Journal of Genetics and Cytology* XVII (3) (Sept. 1975), 297-304.

135. "In Canada, issue is 'kept under wraps'."

136. Dr. Margaret Thompson, geneticist at the Hospital for Sick Children, Toronto, told St. Philip-the-Apostle's parish conference on genetic engineering in Nov. 1973 that one had recently existed in Toronto.

137. In his paper "A.I.D.: asking the right questions," in Archives of the Anglican Church of Canada (Toronto).

138. See M.S. Frankel, *op. cit.*, at footnote 51 supra, on the problems of semen banking.

139. recs. 19 and 21.

140. The reader could usefully consult R.G. Edwards, *op. cit.* in footnote 44 supra, for an introductory survey and bibliography of the subject.

141. I (11) 324-25.

142. Personal communication to Phyllis Creighton by Constance Mungall, researcher for a CBC Ideas program on biomedical advances.

143. A.G. McLaren and M.G. Kerr, "Egg transplantation," *Science Journal* (June 1970), 51-58, at page 56.